New Revised & Updated Edition

Manipulation

The Master Secrets of Covert Persuasion & Hypnotic Influence

By A. Thomas Perhacs

Published by Velocity Group Publishing

PO Box 9516 Hamilton, NJ 08650   www.mindforcesecrets.com

Introduction

DISCLAIMER

Neither A. Thomas Perhacs nor Velocity Group Publishing assumes any responsibility for the use or misuse of the concepts, methods and strategies contained in this book. The reader is warned that the use of some or all of the techniques in this book may result in legal consequences, civil and/or criminal.

USE OF THIS BOOK IS DONE AT YOUR OWN RISK.

(Updated Version, June 2010)

As you begin to read this manual and listen to the audio files, you will start to understand the power this course of instruction can deliver for you.

Many people spend their entire lives trying to find methods, techniques and strategies to make their lives more powerful. Learning how to become more commanding really is an interpretation of what you want to do with this so-called power.

What you will learn is how to not only master yourself better through self-hypnosis, but how you can positively help the people around you. Like all of my courses, this is designed to give you the information that you need without out all of the extra fluff that comes with most books.

I have put together what I feel is the information that you need in order to use these covert persuasion and hypnotic influencing techniques to their maximum.

Many have asked me how I came up with this information and I can tell you that as I started to study Hypnosis, NLP and other Mind Studies back in the late 90's, I realized most books and courses were not laid out in a format where you could learn quickly…

When I started this manuscript, it was designed to be used as my notes for how this works, I had no intention of publishing it on a grand scale or even selling it.

I condensed hundreds of hours of training, thousands of pages of notes and reading into what I consider the Reference Manual to become a highly potent Hypnotic Influencer or Covert Persuasion Expert.

This information is laid out in a manner that you can readily apply it. Immediately you will begin to learn, use and then master these concepts for your own use.

Keep in mind that this manuscript was orginally the work book which accompanies my 8 hour audio course of the same name. You may want to reference the audio files for even more indepth instruction and insights at:

www.mindforcesecrets.com

www.mindforcesecrets.com

These concepts, methods and strategies are designed for informational purposes only and we assume no responsibility for you using this information in the wrong way. That being said, you must understand that with certain levels of supremacy comes the responsibility of using your skills in a responsible manner…

This information is powerful, so just be careful how you use it…

A Thomas Perhacs

Hamilton, New Jersey

June 2010

www.mindforcesecrets.com

Table Of Contents

www.mindforcesecrets.com

www.mindforcesecrets.com

Chapter 1: The Manipulation Factor

What is Manipulation All About?

When I wrote this book, I knew many people would look at the word "Manipulation" as a negative or bad image. My point with using the title "Manipulation" is that no matter what method you use to influence someone, you are manipulating them.

Anytime you convince someone to do something you suggest other than what they want to do, you are in fact manipulating them.

Manipulation: "To Control, Influence or Maneuver"

The word manipulation has several different meanings, some of which may be construed as negative. To be able to manipulate someone or something is not bad in itself, it can only be bad if the intent is to do harm or cause someone problems.

My use of the word manipulation is to be able to do the following:

- To **control** our attitude, beliefs and actions through the autosuggestion and self-hypnosis process
- To be able to **influence** with a degree of strength in order to get someone to come to our way of thinking or doing.
- To be able to **maneuver** someone into an advantages position where the results are a win/win for all parties involved and it is mutually acceptable.

The idea of using your own sense of power to influence someone is as old as our civilization. Without going into all of the history on Hypnosis, Trance Induction, Energy Manipulation, etc (you can look that up on the web), I will try and give you a very easy to understand explanation of what Hypnosis and Trance is and how you can use it to your benefit.

hyp·no·sis (hĭp-nō′sĭs)
n. pl. **hyp·no·ses** (-sēz)

1. An artificially induced altered state of consciousness, characterized by heightened suggestibility and receptivity to direction.

Persuasion & Hypnotic Influence is Like Learning a New Language

As you begin to take the principles in this book and apply them, you are going to have to put in "flight time", which means you will have to log hours in with specific intent to get the desired results of your training.

www.mindforcesecrets.com

Many of the ways you are going to learn to structure your language and sentences may in fact go against how you speak currently. This will cause you to have to stretch your mind to grasp the meaning behind the concepts being taught.

Mental Rehearsal: You Must Be Like an Actor

When an actor performs on stage or in front of a camera, do you think they make up their own lines or do they use a script?

Every actor uses a script to learn their lines. As you begin to learn your lines as it relates to being able to influence or persuade, it is the same thing. You will have to practice your lines over and over (flight time), in order to get the methods and concepts to sink into your mind.

Just like an actor takes on a persona in a role they are doing, you are going to have to do the same exact thing. You will need to step out of your current comfort zone and begin to act ouside of the box.

Get Out of Your Comfort Zone

Everyone has a comfort zone. The goal of this training above all else is the self influence you will achieve in order to pull yourself out of your own comfort zone.

A comfort zone is a place, emotional state where you currently reside in your mind. You need to have the attitude where you are willing to risk a little to receive the maximum benefits of this practice.

The benefits of this will far out weigh any of the resistance you may go through learning it, but this mental preparation is key to getting yourself focused on what you want, not what you don't want.

Begin With The End In Mind

What do you want to be?

Where do you want to go?

Who do you want to be involved with?

What kind of job, business or carreer do you desire?

These and many other questions are what you must ask yourself, so you know what you want out of this situation of Hypnotic Influence and Covert Persuasion.

Set a goal of where you want to be, the kind of skills you want to achieve, and then post a date and work up to it. Once the goal is set, you can then focus on how you are going to get there.

Many have used this training to become Stage Hypnotisits, while others have used these methods to meet someone of the opposite sex. And many more have used these potent concepts to create a lifestyle that resides inside of their mind and allows them to benefit from all areas of their life from their job or business to every relationship they have …

9

Another unique way to think outside of the box is to get a goal and then figure out 10 different ways to get that goal. Write it out on paper and reverse engineer the goal exactly the way you want it to turn out.

That my friends is power!

Becoming a Controller

The true essence of what I am teaching here is showing you how you can become a controller. A controller is the person who is calling the shots in life. If you get nothing but this concept from this book, it will have been worth a hundred times the price you paid…

Being a controller is a mind set based on the facts as you believe them to be not neccesarily what they are currently. Being a controller is a state of mind.

Attitude of a Controller

A controller is the Alpha. He or she is the "Shot Caller" the main man or woman. This is an attitude that you will develop as you begin the process.

Don't ever let a contrary thought in…You are "A Controller". This is what you need to affirm to yourself daily.

"I am in the process of becoming a powerful controller"

"I am the controller in all areas of my life"

Preplay & Rehearse Success

Always set it upon your mind to preplay success. Your subconscious mind is very powerful and you can extract so much more powerful from it than you would ever believe.

It is this belief, that will propell you to your vision of whatever success means to you. The subconscious does what it is used to not what your intent is. This is why you must use repetion to condition it.

Remember and burn into your mind the following two statements:

Controlling Fear

The biggest question I get from people is they are sometimes afraid to try these techniques to see if they will work. After all, we are doing a lot of this covertly, so it makes sense you will sometimes be hesitant with a new technique or method.

Keep in mind what was said before about being an actor. You have to get into your role to make yourself comfortable at times. Remember this when controlling fear of the unknown.

" It is not the lack of fear, but the overcoming of fear"

And how do you do that?

www.mindforcesecrets.com

By taking action. The more action you take, the more the fear will subside. Everyone has fear, it is just getting focused on the goal ahead.

All Learning is State Dependent

Anytime you learn something, it is dependent on what kind of state you are in at the time. If you learn that touching a hot stove gets you a burn, you have learned a valuable lesson.

Anytime after that, when you get near a hot stove, your mind will automatically remind you of that state, and you will keep your hands clear from the stove.

We learn from our:

- Physiology

- Emotional States

So that means in order to grasp certain concepts, if you can put yourself into a phsyiological state as another time you learned something or the same emotiional state, then it stands to reason you can learn that thing that much quicker.

Using Energy to Get to Desired States

This topic will sound strange to many of you and to some you may not even believe it, but I can tell you from first hand experience as well as from those of many people over the years, who have used energy alone to create a desired state within someone.

I won't go into my seminar on intrinsic energy, but I will mention, that your energy can be used so much more powerfully than you could ever even imagine.

Here a few ways to mentally use your energy to get someone into a desired state.

- Throw an energy ball

- Project energy directly at them

- Project an energetic intent

- Project an image or a thought

When your mind conjures up an image, that image can be transferred to another person. If you are good at visualizing this can be accomplished quite easlly.

I have known many who have used this projection technique in order to get someone into a desired state.

Example: The best state or emotional energy you would want someone to be in would be happy, open minded, euphorice, blissful. Anytime you can send those types of thoughts or energy to someone, you will get terrific results.

www.mindforcesecrets.com

Every Thought Gets Sent Out To "Neuro-Transmitters"

Everytime you think, it creates a transmission of energy that gets sent out to our "Neuro-Transmitters (Brain Recepters and receivers).

So in essence, what that means is that your subconscious mind receives every thought another person thinks. The only thing is, can you actually decode the transmission.

The subconscious does in fact decode and receive all messages, that is why subliminal suggestions work so well, because the subconscious receives them all.

That doesn't mean that all suggestions will be acted upon. It depends on how you construct the suggestion or message (See Chapter 6)

> **"Some of the most powerful influence will be done by Subconscious Non-Verbal Communication"**

Using An Energetic Compression

To receive even better results, you can use an Energtic Compression Mechanism which will allow you to imbed the energy even better. Here are several ways to use this.

- **Moved Energy**- This is directly related to the prementioned items on energy

- **Physical Gestures/Movements**- Just by using a certain gesture someone can tell what you are thinking about.

- **Sound**- Any sound that could construe a certain emotion- bordom, excitement, etc.

- **Visualization**- Similar to above referenced

- **Posture**- Your posture gives away a lot. Stand tall, erect, strong versus slouched or lazy looking.

All of these portray a picture and that picture or energy can be sent or received from someone. You can send it out as the actual representation or you could send it out to deceive someone as if to give them a fals sense of your true energy and ability.

Professional Hypnotic Persuaders Create a Web of Powerful Suggestions of:

- Feelings

- Actions

- Thought Processes

The Difference Between Men and Women

There is a definate difference in how the sexes can be influenced or persuaded. The differences are absolutely accurate and as we go through this training, you will really want to make a mental note of

www.mindforcesecrets.com

this, because it will really allow you to understand how to use certain techniques on women and different ones on men.

Men: Are vulnerable to visual representations. Most men are visual and will react very well to the visual. Think about it this way. Men really get excited when they see a good looking woman. That is visual.

Women: Are much more vulnerable to language and words. That is why you can sway a woman much more easily by building word pictures and using very descriptive language. Some women might not find a man attractive, but by speaking with him, if he uses descriptive or romantic "type" of words, the woman will become attracted.

Relaxation-Comfort-Confidence

Here again is a very potent combination which can be used to manipulate someone. Get them relaxed, get them comfortable and build a confidence in yourself with the person, and you are about 80-90% of the way there. This is without ever using a hypnotic type of command or structure.

> **"What ever you put serious effort in, your subconscious believes"**

> **"Conviction doesn't come from mental rehearsal but by physical experience"**

www.mindforcesecrets.com

Chapter 2: Into The Mind of Trance

Into The Mind

Most people view Hypnosis or an altered state of consciousness to be something that is mysterious and hidden, a skill that only a magician or some guy wearing a cape with a pendulum that swings back and forth as he summons you with, "look at the swinging object as you go into a deep sleep". This is a valid technique, but one that you will learn to use just as effectively. Cape must be purchased seperately.

These types of concepts work well and we will touch on why this works and how you can get it to work, but what we are going to be discussing is how to pull off a Hypnotic Trance while just talking to someone in a normal everyday conversation.

The Central Rule of Mental Power

> "He/She who knows and uses the laws of suggestion protects himself from all worries and achieves all that he/she desires/"

Conversational Hypnotic Influence

So, how do we hypnotize someone when we are mearly speaking with them? The fact of the matter is you put people into a mild trance anytime you speak with them and they are actually following your words intently.

How can this be possible?

Anytime someone focuses on you while you are speaking, and allows themselves to get involved in your story, they are actually going into a light trance. Now on the other hand, if you are speaking with someone and they are pre-occupied or not focusing on what you are saying, they are in a different kind of trance. They are in a self-trance as they focus on whatever they are currently thinking about.

Have you ever noticed someone who you were talking to, but you knew they weren't listening to you, they were just waiting for their turn to speak? This is someone in a self-trance.

Trance & Strength of Concentration

Strength of Concentration is really what Trance is all about. Throughout most of the day, we go in and out of trance. Our mind is divided into two very distinct but connected sections, the Conscious and Sub-Conscious portions of the mind:

www.mindforcesecrets.com

Conscious Mind: This is the intentional or deliberate mind. When you actively think about something you are using your conscious mind. The conscious mind sometimes will get in your way because it sometimes bases things on what it perceives as logical.

Sub-Conscious Mind: This is the part of the mind below the level of conscious perception. Unlike the conscious mind basing itself on logic, the sub-conscious (or unconscious Mind) will accept all information that is introduced to it.

Have you ever seen someone watching TV that was so into the program that when you spoke to them, they didn't answer? This person was in a trance in front of the TV. That television program would be influencing this person tremendously. Here is a partial list of some of the times you go into a self- inflicted trance:

- While watching television, listening to the radio or a music CD
- While driving a car
- Day dreaming
- When someone is telling you a story and because of the content, it takes your thoughts off into a different direction.

These are very potent trance states that are developed everyday by everyone. A trance is really as simple as that.

Trance: Changing the emotional state that someone is in and using that state to influence them by making powerful, controlled suggestions to their subconscious mind.

As you start to learn how to use the concepts of putting someone into a trance, you will find there will be primarily three stages of trance depth that someone can go into. We will primarily be concerned with a light trance, as most of the trance work we will be doing is through a conversational tone.

The Three Levels of Trance

1. **Hypnoid** - Light trance with eyes fluttering
2. **Cataleptic** - Eyes go side to side
3. **Somnambulistic** - Deep trance where eyes role up. The personally is generally relaxed and is a "sleep like" state.

Because trance is so much a part of what we do every day, there are many ways that you can actually induce a trance in yourself and others. One of the keys to becoming good at hypnotic influencing and being able to increase the suggestibility of others is to learn how to put yourself into a trance.

The fact is there are probably 30 levels of trance, but why go into all that, when you really only need to know how to put someone in a trance.

The basics of putting someone into a trance is to learn how to change their state. If someone were in one state, you would want to move them into another, thus causing a light trance, due to their having to make an effort to switch to a different state.

www.mindforcesecrets.com

Example: If you had someone in a happy or upbeat mood and you made them angry, like in a road rage incident, you would change their state, thus causing them to be much more likely to be put into a very deep state of trance...

> **"A rule of thumb is that the quicker and deeper you can get yourself into a trance like state the quicker you will be able to get others into it."**

Going Deeper Into Trance

You will hear a lot of hypnotists talking about going into trance deeper and deeper. This is common, and there are many ways that you can get yourself into a trance and also the person that you are hypnotizing or persuading.

The following are some ways to induce a trance like effect on yourself and others

- **Staring at an object**- This is the focusing method that is so common among hypnotists and for good reason, it works. Anytime you transfix your gaze on any one object, as your eyes focus on the object, your consciousness starts to dig into the moment, thus causing you to be able to be influenced greater.
- **Candles**- Candles are less well known, but add another level of sophistication to the trance because they give off an energy as well as the light. This allows you to go even deeper into trance.
- **Incense**- This gives you the olfactory concentration. Why do you think mystics use candles and incense? It is not just for the look. They both carry essential powerful components, which allow things to happen.
- **Music**- There is certain music, when listened to, can take you into a light trance. Combine this with an induction or some of the other mentioned tools and the trance could become quite deep.
- **Hypnotic Posters and Devices**- These devices are very rare and few know about them, but they are by far the most powerful of the aforementioned. These devices are specifically designed to induce a trance. They are extremely strong and should be used with caution.

Trance Strategies

Here are some tips to get your trances to work even better and to be more effective.

- Change their state and they will go into trance
- Go into the state first yourself- Some states
  - Buying
  - Excitement
  - Desire
  - Something to do
- Use confusion- Interrupt their current thought process

Confusion is your friend when you are looking to put someone in a trance. A common way to do this is to interrupt their current thought process thus allowing you to change their state. Take someone

16

www.mindforcesecrets.com

that is angry and get them to a state of laughter and it not only breaks their current state, but gives you a doorway into their mind.

- Ask them questions that cause them to process the answer
    - How do you feel about?
    - How did you feel about?
    - Wouldn't you?
    - Aren't You?
    - Don't You?
    - Isn't it?
- Tell a story that is very difficult to follow and has trance words, commands and other mechanisms built right in. We will cover this in detail in another chapter.

Utilize Everything Around You

This principle is a powerful one and understanding it could mean the difference between getting these concepts to work or not. When learning how to persuade someone to do what you would like for him or her to do, you need to be able to utilize every type of stimulus that you can to get them involved in the process, such as:

- **Noise:** Using noises to allow them to become aware of what is going on around them.
    - **Example-** " As you listen to the sound of the traffic, you will get more relaxed and go deeper into an excellent feeling"

- **Objection:** As they object to you, you use that objection to turn them around
    - **Example-** " So you don't find me that attractive. The more you find me not that attractive, the more you will find me all the more attractive because you will begin to see my other qualities and they will cause you to see me as attractive in another way".

- **Trance:** The ability to change someone's internal or external state will enable you to put them into a trance. The level of trance depends on how much you work on it.
    - **Example-** " As you just listen to what I have to say, you will start to feel really good about us working together, and as you reflect on what I say you will begin to feel even better about us working together"

- **Feelings:** People are driven by feelings. The more you can tap into their feelings the more you can get people to act. We are all very emotional and are driven by feelings of some sort or the other be they feelings of love, power, sensual ness, happiness, sadness, etc.
    - **Example-** Once you begin to feel the power of what this course will bring to you, you will be able to see how that will cause you to feel even more powerful.

More Advanced Methods of Trancing

Hypnosis is in essence is the ability to put someone in a trance. I like to call it a "trance like state", because it is more relevant for what we are actually doing…

As you begin to understand this process, you will use some of these methods and others you may never use. It comes down to comfort level and what works best for your personality and the way you think.

Expert Trancing Revealed

As with cooking, when you have the right recipe, with the right ingredients, you can make a wonderful dish. Well, the same is true when getting someone into trance.

These are the very same methods professional hypnotists and controllers use day in and day out to gain control of someone's mind. Here is a list of concepts to work on.

- Relaxation

- Changing Their State

- Interrupting Their State

- Emotional Ploy

- Closing The Eyes

- Hypnotic Devices

- Eye Fascination

- Sound and Light increases the trance

- Add Kinestetics to the Visualization process

  - Feel it

  - See it

  - Be it

How Do You Know The Trance is Working?

The easiest way to tell if the trance is working is did they respond to your suggestions. One of the keys to getting feedback from the trance subject is to ask questions, that when answered properly will allow you to know if they are going or are already in the trance…

Again the trance is a shifting of one state to a more focused one. Very similar to when you are day dreaming or even whille driving your car.

How many times while driving your car have you day dreamed and missed an exit or suddenly noticed you were 20 miles out of your way because of the hypnotic day dream trance state that your mind took you on?

www.mindforcesecrets.com

The Induction By Interruption Technique

This famous technique is one of the easiest ways to test your ability to get someone into trance fast. This one technique can be modified once you understand the underlying principles of this very effective technique…

This can be used as you shake someone's hand. As your subject comes over to you to shake your hand, as they grasp your hand lift theirs up in front of their face you command that they concentrate on their hand.

As they do describe what they can see in their hand and tell them to, "go into trance only as slowly as your arm begins to drift down to your side"

At this they will begin to lower their arm and as they do, because they are staring at their hand, their eyes will also begin to close. As their arm continues to drift down suggest to them that, "as your hand touches against your leg you will instantly go deep into trance, deeper and deeper into trance".

 As soon as they have done this tell them to only pay attention to the sound of your voice and continue with a deepening script such as the ones which are included in the induction section of this book.

www.mindforcesecrets.com

Chapter 3: Self Hypnosis & Auto-Suggestions

What is Self Hypnosis?

Self-Hypnosis is the process of putting yourself into trance so that you can effect change within yourself. It is a very common practice and may go by many different names. Many athletes use the power of self-suggestion to psyche themselves up before a competition. This is a form of Self-Hypnosis.

Self-Hypnosis is getting your strength of concentration to a point where you become very focused on whatever you are doing at the time. You can use many of the same methods you used for trance to get you the results you need with self-hypnosis.

Autosuggestions

Autosuggestion is the science of using affirmations or suggestions to influence the subconscious mind. Very much like self hypnosis, except that autosuggestions are designed to implant very direct suggestions into the subconscious mind.

The difference is self hypnosis is the act of putting yourself in a trance. Once there you can decide how to use the self hypnosis. When you combine autosuggestions with the self hypnosis, it makes it so much more powerful than when used just by itself.

In Napoleon Hill's best selling book, **Think and Grow Rich**, Autosuggestion is covered in great detail and as a matter of fact, it is described in a very easy to understand way.

Using Autosuggestions for Others

You can also use Autosuggestions as a means to influence others. Anytime you think a thought, you transmit a thought. When you take these thoughts and place them in a logical trajectory, the can then become suggestions you will use to influence people at a distance.

For example, if we were talking to one another and I mearly thought of a suggestion and directed it directly into your mind, this would be a form of autosuggestion.

> **"Autosuggestions can be used for self or to be implanted into the mind of another. This one concept is a secret of Covert Persuasion".**

Some Keys to Self Hypnosis

Entire books have been written on how to effectively Self Hypnotize. My goal is to make it simple for you. Here are some great tips for your success with self hypnosis.

www.mindforcesecrets.com

Here are some keys to Self-Hypnosis

- It must be done on a regular basis
- All references must be made in the first person- " I am a highly successful and prosperous person", "My body is relaxing deeper and deeper into a state of warmth and comfort"
- The key is to relax the body down
- Everything must be positive

Being In The Process

To take your autosuggestions to an even higher and more powerful level, one secret which can be worth a fortune to you is adding these simple words, "In The Process".

Think about this: When you give your mind a direction, it takes many times before it actually will act on that suggestion in the way you want it to.

If you say to your subconscious: " I am a millionaire", it will more than likely reject that statement because it knows it isn't true. Now if you repeat it enough and get the mind to accept it then you have done a great job. But why work so hard when there is an easier way…

If using autosuggestions work, then why wouldn't that statement work?

The reason is because it is too big a stretch to go from the known (where you are) to the unknown (where you want to go). That is why you want to use the following statement on many of your self auto suggestions.

"I am in the process to becoming a millionaire"

Sounds simple, but think about it. When you are in the process, the mind can't refute it. The mind must process the directive like any other directive you tell it.

When you state "you are", the mind can take a selective choice on if you are telling the truth or not. By using "In The Process", you will get must faster results than any other method of self talk.

This is such a secret because most don't know it. This one idea is priceless, if you will use it to get the results you are striving for.

> **"Being in the process is so much easier for the subconscious mind to digest and will exponentially increase your autosuggestions"**

21

Using a Self Hypnosis Induction to Implant Autosuggestions

Remember that you can use the following induction with your own affirmations and goals. You can also use any type of visualzation that you like as well. You may also focus on your third eye or work on your remote sensing and out of body skills as well.

Self Hypnosis Induction (Record This to Play back)

Simply use this induction script and record it to place on your Ipod or CD to get the most benefits from this. Repitition is a key and this should be used several times per day.

"I am sitting down, eyes closed, relaxed...My arms and legs are flexible...I am quite relaxed... Nothing can distract me... I am quite calm... I let myself be drawn along. I am breathing slowly, regularly... I am feeling quite well... A pleasant peacefulness envelops my body"

" I will take a deep breath and while exhaling will exhale all tension, stress and negativity in my life. It wil go away and I will feel refreshed and energized.

"Now, I am concentrating on my facial muscles... My cheek muscles are growing heavy, totally relaxed. My jaw muscles are totally relaxing down.... I am relaxing the muscles in my forehead and they are getting quite heavy... My entire facial area is relaxing down. My eyelids are heavy... Heavier and heavier... My eyes are hermetically closed... I can no longer open them... I no longer want to... My neck muscles are now relaxing down, I feel a comfort and relaxation throughout my head and neck.... Now I am concentrating on my torso, including my chest, back, stomach and all of my internal organs. These areas are now relaxing down.. ... My entire torso is relaxed... Feels heavy as if being drawn downward.... My arms are growing heavy... They are drawn downward... This heaviness prevades my arms more and more... More and more... Now, my arms are as heavy as lead. I am concentrating on my legs... I am quite calm... I clearly feel them growing heavy... More and more.... Now, my legs are quite heavy. As heavy as lead. I let myself sink more and more into this wonderful feeling of relaxation and heaviness... I am more and more relaxed... More and more relaxed"

"With each exhale my body goes deeper and deeper into this state of relaxation and heaviness. I will now teach my body to relax down even more.... I will countdown from 3-1 and I will get more relaxed with each count... I will go deeper with each count.

www.mindforcesecrets.com

3……….I am going ten times deeper than the moment before;

2………. I am going twenty times deeper than the moment before;

1………. I am going one hundred times deeper than the moment before.

"Nothing can distract me… I hear only my voice… I feel myself sinking still more, more and more deeply into this feeling of peace… I feel quite well… I am sinking deeper and deeper… More and more."

"Every cell, in every part of my body, has now risen to a higher state of power… Is glowing like a high-energy dynamo… Is giving off magnetism and energy that turns others irresistibly towards me… That pulls what I want and what I need out of my surroundings.

"My body is now surrounded by this invisible field of physical magnetism and energy… It never tires… It never dims… It is always there to protect me… To draw to me what I want… I have the self-confidence I have always dreamed of… I can now make my dreams become my realities… I have the power to do this because God has blessed me with this power…"

- *I have total faith and belief in my ability to control all areas in my life, based on the power with which God has blessed me;*

- *I am disciplined & stay focused on my goals;*

- *I am relaxed and in control at all times;*

- *I am a positive influence on everyone with whom I come in contact;*

- *I expect success every day;*

- *I am bold and confident;*

- *I keep my thoughts pure and good, and channel my energy into creative, worthwhile actions;*

- *My mind is strong and I achieve all of my goals and objectives on time.*

- *I am in the process of earning (amount) per month/year.*

- ***I am in the process of weighing a strong an healthy (number of pounds)***

"I will use this power wisely... It will help others at the same time it helps me... I will do no harm with it... It is too great to misuse... I will employ it for good only... For my good... and for the good of the world...

" When I come out of this state of relaxation I will feel as if I have been sleeping for several hours, fully refreshed and ready to take on any challenges and activities that the day holds."

Self Hypnosis is a Process

You may have to Self Hypnotize yourself often in order to get the suggestions to properly implant inside of your subcionscious. We go into much more detail in the Closed Door Hypnosis Total Control Files book, which is specifically desinged for Self Hypnosis and Auto-Suggestion Mastery.

www.mindforcesecrets.com

Chapter 4: Bonding & Rapport

Establishing Rapport at a Strong Level

Rapport: *Is the ability to create a bond with someone that you meet.*

This could be for business or pleasure, but the key is to get someone to start to feel comfortable when they are around you. Generally, you will be able to influence someone after you have gotten them to:

- **Know You**
- **Like You**
- **Trust You**

Likes In Bonding

Did you ever go to an office building or a business meeting where everyone was dressed in suits and ties? Of course you have, and this shows you exactly the process of being "like". The old saying, **"When in Rome, do as the Romans do"** absolutely applies when it comes to this type of technology.

Rapport can be developed many different ways and we are going to cover several. If you've ever heards of the statement that "opposites attract", it is the most rediculous statement ever made, because from all of the data I have "likes attract". Have you ever seen a situation where "opposites actually attracted"?

That being said, lets learn how we can create a bond with people the instant we meet them, shall we?

How do you get someone to know you, like you and trust you in a very short period of time? By getting in rapport with them in a way that literally forces them to know, like and trust you.

Modeling for Quick Rapport and Bonding

Modeling is the concept that we try to be as much like someone as possible to immediately allow them to consciously and even more important unconsciously see us as "just like them"

So much has been written about this, but I am going to break this down in the easiest way I know, so you can get it to work for you as quickly as possible.

Check this out. We are going to model the person in a most unique way…

25

Mirroring Methods For Rapid Rapport Building

We are going to get into rapport quickly by modeling the person in several different ways:

- **Physical:** We match what they do by using a mirroring effect. This could include but not be limited to the way they carry themselves, how they sit, their facial gestures, eye movements, breathing, etc.
    - o **Example-** They Cross Their arms- I do the same

- **Verbal (match words):** We say back to them what they say in the way that they say it causing a familiarity with them.
    - o **Example-** They use a phrase- I use it also (but artfully)

- **Pace mood, belief, opinion:** As you become more sensitive to someone's feelings you can start to pick up on their mood and then direct yourself to get into their mood and then slowly bring them into your mood.
    - o **Example-** They have an opinion- You agree, get into deeper rapport and then you can start to influence them to your way of thinking.

- **Intent:** You go into the situation intending for that person to really start to bond with you.
    - o **Example-** You go into the situation knowing beforehand that they absolutely want to get to know you better.
- **Breathing:** You follow their breathing pattern and then get on the same breathing pattern as them.
    - o **Example-** Notice how they are breathing in and out and start to get into the same breathing rate. This powerful method is the hardest to do, but when mastered gets you into rapport the quickest.

Once you get into rapport with someone, you will be able to influence them much greater than if you were to try some of the other techniques without it.

Once you get into rapport with them by either mirroring or matching what they are doing, you can then begin to bring them over to what you are doing so that you will now be leading the rapport process.

Entire courses are taught on Rapport alone, and these concepts will allow you to get to bond with people much quicker. Keep in mind that all of the methods contained here take a lot of practice and effort to get good at them.

Posturing For Success- Using Disarming Questions

Once in rapport you can begin to create the bond by taping into their mind by asking them questions that allow you to move the conversation in any direction you want. Here are a couple right off, but I will provide many more by the time we are done.

- is it okay to sit here and begin'?
- I'm wondering?
- I asked myself
- I'm curious...

Personality Types

As your developing rapport, most people have personality traits that if you are aware, will allow you to interpret your strategy to persuade and influence them.

There are four listed and what you will find is that most people are a combination of these types. What you need to do is listen, look and understand where they are, because the sooner you understand where they are coming from the sooner, you can influence them.

Sharks: These are highly motivated type "A" personality. Probably money motivated, works long hours, doesn't mess around. Probably is a fast talker. An example would be a New Yorker. Very fast paced, get things done type of person.

Dolphins: These people just want to have fun. They enjoy life to the fullest; so don't rain on their parade. Probably don't take things to serious. An example could be someone from California.

Whales: These folks like to help people. They are kind and considerate. They want to make sure things go right. Very slow talker. Always looking for someone else's best interest. An example might be someone from the South-Georgia.

Urchins: These are the analytical person. Just want the facts. Analyze everything you say. Very skeptical. "I'll see it before I believe it" type of person. This person could be from the MidWest-Wisconsin.

Visual-Auditory-Kinesthetic Strategy

This is a very important strategy that is used in the use of Covert Persuasion and Hypnotic Influencing, and is really an important part of the entire process in getting someone to come to your way of thinking. The VAK Representational systems are an integral strategy in order to begin to influence with Power.

www.mindforcesecrets.com

All of us represent things in a truly unique and personal way. Some of us refer to things in a very visual way and some of us use more of an auditory or kinesthetic reference point. The importance here is being able to recognize where someone's representational systems are so that you can begin to add those reference points into your influence and persuasion skills.

The key to this entire process is building rapport with power and to do this you need to add as many tricks as you can to the situation. Once you get their representational system down, you can then start to add scenarios that will fulfill what it is that they relate to.

Visual: This represents the person that sees things from a visual viewpoint. This comes out in the way they speak often times with sayings such as, "I see what you mean" and "Look how I can help you".

Auditory: From the auditory viewpoint a person represents phrases such as "Do you hear what I am saying?" or "That idea rings a bell with me".

Kinesthetic: These are the people that are touchy feely and like the physical contact and use this in their representational systems, such as, "That is a hot idea" or "That song really touches me".

Once you understand someone's representational system you can then start to use that in your persuasion and communication with them. The benefit is you will gain deeper rapport and get the abiltiy to influence them even deeper because now you are more like them because of your use of rapport techniques and modeling their own VAK System

www.mindforcesecrets.com

Chapter 5: Setting The Hypnotic Game Plan

What is Your Game Plan?

Setting up your ability to Hypnotically Influence and Persuade Covertly all comes down to setting up a game plan that works. I have set up all the concepts for you to be successful, all you have to do is implement them…

I am going to cover in this chapter some of the most powerful concepts in the entire Hypnotic Influence and Covert Persuasion arsenal.

Reasons/Intents/Challenges

This could be the single most important aspect of influence and persuasion, because it allows you to find out exactly what will influence this person to take action. It also includes using two very important strategies that will allow you dig deep into what the person really wants, needs and is motivated by.

> **"Everyone does something for a specific reason or intent. Once you find out what their reasons and intents are, you can figure out a way to present the solution to their challenge"**

Finding Out Challenges

When you can find out what someone's challenges are, you can find out how you can help them come up with solutions to their challenges.

Example:

"While I realize that you don't yet know a lot about me, let me just pose something to you. (Name), If I were to ask you…. What's the one aspect of what you do that is a challenge or that you find most fulfilling, either because you have to find the right people or software or you just have to focus in to get yourself motivated to do it, what would that be?"

Once you find out what their challenges are you then use that to strategically use your persuasion skills (presuppositions, trances, embedded commands, etc).

www.mindforcesecrets.com

Reasons/Intents

This is one of the best formulas to get people to tell you exactly what they want. This method is so powerful that it works even without the use of the other strategies.

- What's significant about...
- What's behind that?
- Because'?
- So, ultimately what would this mean to you?
- What would you do with *"ultimate reason"1*

Moving Towards or Away

Finding out what motivates a person in terms of, are they someone that goes toward goals or moves away from difficulties. This strategy lets you know how to represent your patterns to them and tie in whether they are moving toward or away.

Moving Towards: This is the type of person that views things from a positive position and is always looking ahead and looking for the future.

Example: Someone who looks at their job as a bridge to the future. Someone that will take some risks to get there.

Moving Away: This person views things from more of the negative perspective.

Example: They look at their job as their security and their view is to do a good job and not look to lose it.

The reason you want to know this is how to influence them more powerfully. It is also important not to use "going towards" types of methods for someone that is a "moving away" person. If you do this you will break rapport and not be able to influence quite as well.

What will having *"reasons"* do for you?

The Power of Your Presence

When I talked about you becoming a Controller, I really meant it. This one factor will increase your chances to become good at this over all other skills.

You need to carry yourself with power. You need to walk in a room and expect everyone to turn around to face you. Your presence preceeds you and allows you the benefits of those without that presence.

Another concept you need to embrace is the concept of being comfortable with power. Take that concept and breath it in deep. The power is all around you. It eminates from your being...

Please understand that the power I am referring to is a self-power that allow you to conquer all fear and become the person you desire to be.

30

This power is not a power that usurps someone else, but one that feels good to others. It is a comfort of power, a euphoric feeling that only one that has the power can transmit to someone.

You are that person, now embrace it!

Subconscious Non-Verbal Communication

There are three levels to your communication

- What You say verbally

- What you say mentally

- What your energy says

These 3 powerful concepts are extremely potent when used together. When you are a controller, you use all three of these types of communication at the same time.

Now, this will take some time getting used to using all three forms at the same time. Let me provide an example:

I command you- "The more you hear the sound of my voice, the more powerful you will feel"

I think to you- You are feeling more and more powerful

I send you an energy of power that feels extraordinary.

I know I keep saying that this is powerful and that is powerful, but once you begin to grasp the potency of techniques in your hands you will finally come to realize the true power that you can weild...

The Power of Tonality

While I am speaking about power, lets bring up the concept of your voice and the tones you emit. Your voice is one of the most powerful aspects of your presence.

It will take time to get your voice to the place you need it to be, but once you do, look out, you will be a killer when it comes to persuading and influencing.

Everytime you speak, a tone is emitted along with an energy. That energy is controlled by you. When you speak you can choose how you want your words to come out and depending on who you are speaking to makes a difference in the tone you will use.

Hard Raspy Tone: This is a tone for a powerful male. Not one you would use in front of a female. This tone can be soothing, yet at the same time commanding. (See audios for examples)

Soft Tone: The soft tone is lilting in the way you speak it. Used for woman and children. This tone soothes those that hear it. Children are comforted by it and women are wooed by it.

Many times, the soft tone can be used as an empahsis of a command as well. Again power is in your voice, use it wisely.

31

      www.mindforcesecrets.com

The Power of Your Eyes

When you combine the eyes with the power of your voice, you have a complete double whammy effect on the person you are looking to influence…

There is really power that comes from the eyes. There is a reason why "The eyes are the windows to the soul". This statement is so true and you must begin to use your eyes to your own advantage…

Have you ever noticed how a woman can bat their eyes and get results?

Just look in a mirror and notice the different types of energy that form out of your eyes as you:

- Make a gesture of shock

- Make a gesture of happiness

- Look angry

- Look pleased

This power that emenates can be used very effectively with your non-verbal communication and should be one of the key focuses for your training.

Now there are two main differences in eye power that you need to be made aware of :

- **Soft Eyes**- Soft eyes are the mode you will want to use the majority of the time. The energy is pleasing and will allow you to be more covert in your communication. Soft eyes can be done by closing the eyes slghtly as if they are "half open". This mutes the energy, and combined with you thinking of a pleasant energy coming out of your eyes, works quite well.

- **Strong Eyes**- These "blazing" eyes emit a lot of power, but in most cases, it will be too much for someone to handle (subconsciously). This focused stair can be used effectively with someone else with a strong personality, or someone who knows you are going to control them (as in a formal induction).

Practice with your eye power, and I can promise you will start to see amazing results.

Using Your Hands As Transmitters

The hands can be very powerful as it relates to energy and hypnotic power. You can direct your hands in a way which causes your subject to follow your every word.

This takes some time getting used to, but the hands can be used in so many different ways. When you use your hands to emphasize a point, the subject often times follows the hands. When they do this, just like they were looking at a pendulum swinging back and forth, they begin to become somewhat tranced out.

The better control you have with your hands the more powerful you will become in regards to hypnotising someone without them even knowing it.

Make a pass across someone with your hands and you will notice their eyes following the direction of your pass. This method has been used for years by hypnotists and controllers alike.

The key to this is to not over use it by "talking with your hands". The hands can be an emphasis that projects energy and intent, not just wildly flailing about while you talk.

Power Systems For You

Keep in mind that the information covered in this chapter is imperative for you to get your techniques to work. Without the proper mental focus as well as your ability to use your hands, voice and eyes, you won't be as effective as a "Controller".

A controller is someone who knowlingly uses all the tools in their tool box in order to get a specifically intended result. By utilizing the concepts in this chapter, you will have more power than anyone else using techniques without these concepts.

So many today discount the energetic side of Hypntoic Influence. This in effect is your advantage. Use the energy you have through your intent and presence and you will be amazed with the results. Combine the eyes, voice and hands and you will be on your way to becoming a potent "Controller"

www.mindforcesecrets.com

Chapter 6: Subliminal Suggestions & Messages

What Exactly is a Subliminal Message

A Subliminal Message is a technique for "planting" a thought (state, process, or experience) within the mind of another person beneath the person's conscious awareness.

This is done through many different techniques including but not limited to *presuppositions*, which are assumptions implied within verbal structures.

Do Sublminal Messages Really Work?

The concept of subliminal messsages has been around for as long as time. The thing is, people use subliminal suggestions even without knowing it. I guess I should break the subliminal formats down so you understand them better

- **Messages**- The message can be a reference or sending information to someone. Used in advertising all of the time. Can be subtle yet powerful method. Anytime you imply something it sinks directly into the subconscious for verification.

- **Suggestions**- Similar to the message, but the difference is it suggests an outcome more specifically.

- **Commands**- These are direct commands to the subconscious with overt directions. "You will do this or that"

As stated before, the reason subliminal messages work is because the subconscious takes in all of the information you send to it and processes it. If you are skilled enough to parse that information in the form of a speicific directive of you're choosing, then you are able to influence at the highest level.

Subliminal Embedded Commands

Rather than giving instructions directly, you can embed directives within a larger sentence structure. These powerful methods are how you influence their subconscious mind indirectly similar to subliminal influence.

*"You can begin to **<u>relax.</u>**"*

*"I don't know how soon you'll **<u>feel better</u>**."*

Throughout the remainder of this manual and course, you will notice that all of the subliminal commands are in bold, underlined for effect. I want you to use this method anytime you are setting up a sentence to be used, so you can get familiar with each part of the message.

We are also going to talk about embedded commands which are contained in a sentence structure for maximum effectiveness. The embedded command will be set up with a "pattern" or suggestive statement that elicits a specific response.

We will be using certain phrases to set up the command, so it can be successfully implanted into the mind of the subject. This is why this is covert. We are not telling them ahead of time, that we will be implanting the thought, message, command, etc. This is some of the most covert communication you will be taught.

The purpose of using embedded commands is to move your subjects mind in the direction you want it to go without seeming to be intruding or commanding them to do so

When you embed directives within a larger sentence, you can deliver them more smoothly and gracefully, and the listener will not consciously realize that directives have been given. The above messages are likely to have a much more graceful impact than if you were to give the directives alone: **"Relax." "Feel better."**

Marking The Directive

Subliminal and embedded commands are particularly powerful when used with a mechanism that marks out the directive more strongly. This means that you set the directive apart from the rest of the sentence with some nonverbal behavior.

You could do this by:

- **Raising the volume of your voice when delivering the directive**
- **Pausing before and after the directive**
- **Changing your voice tone**
- **Gesturing with one of your hands**
- **Raising your eyebrows.**

You can use any behavior that is perceptible to the other person to mark out a directive for special attention. The other person does not need to notice your marking consciously; in fact they will often respond more fully when your marking is perceived but not consciously recognized.

Three Phases

1. **Soon Something Will Happen**- As you listen to the sound of my voice you will (set command)

2. **You Are Feeling It Happen**- You are Becoming more and more excited about this.

3. **Now It's Happened**- You are excited about this.

Using Commands

Commands are exactly what it says, commands. Think of it this way. What ever you desire as an outcome that is the command you will want to use.

www.mindforcesecrets.com

A simple way to think of it is if you went up to someone and said.

"Give me $100".

"Go out with me"

Now, of course it is not that easy, but in essence it really is, because when you do it covertly, your message is getting across as if you just blatently said those commands to someone.

See the next page for an good list of commands to start off with.

- Trust Me
- Allow Me
- Believe Me
- Buy now
- See the Benefits
- Experience the Value
- I Can Help You
- Act on My Advice
- Follow My Lead
- Make This Happen
- Feel Real Good
- Come to the Conclusion
- This is For You
- Start to Realize
- Make the Decision
- Discover the Value
- Get Excited
- Anticipate the Benefits

- Hire Me
- You Will Want To
- Make This Automatic
- Adopt This Style
- Be Compelled
- Learn More
- Studies Show That
- Most People Would Agree
- (Person of Influence) Said That
- Open up Your Mind
- I Will Immediately Help You
- Become Aware
- Understand the Value
- You Are Thrilled
- Take Action
- Believe Strongly

www.mindforcesecrets.com

Embedded Questions

Questions, like commands, can be embedded within a larger sentence structure.

"I'm curious to know *what you would like to gain from this course*?"

"I'm wondering *what you would like to do next to move this process along?*"

Typically people will respond to the embedded question in the first example, **"What would you like to gain from this course?"** without realizing that the question was not asked directly. The listener doesn't refuse to answer the question, because it is embedded within a statement about the speaker's curiosity. This provides a very gentle and graceful way to gather information.

Negative Commands

When a command is given in its negative form, the positive instruction is generally what is responded to.

For example, if someone says ***"Don't* think of the color red"** you have to think of the color red to understand the sentence. Negation does not exist in primary experience of sights, sounds, and feelings.

Negative commands can be used effectively by stating what you *do* want to occur and preceding this statement with the word "don't."?

"I *don't* want you to **feel** too **comfortable**."

"Don't **have** too much **fun** doing this."

Generally the listener will respond by experiencing what it's like to feel comfortable or to have fun doing this as a way of understanding the sentence.

Dropping The Message Into the Subconscious

In the next chapter, I will go into great detail on some of the patterns and how they work and why they work so well. Let me just give you a simple formula in order to get the process of Suliminal Messaging working for you.

> **Suggestive Phrase + Command + Presence/Energy/Tonality = Subliminal Message**

www.mindforcesecrets.com

So, in essence it's like taking one piece adding another, then another and you get the basis for your commands to be placed sublimnally in the subjects mind. It's a very simple recipe for success.

It really is that simple, and yet most people make it more complicated than it sounds. Remember when I mentioned putting in the right amount of "Fight Time"? Well that is the real key to getting this to work extremely well.

Just like an actor, you must rehearse your lines over and over again. The first time you do this you will probably screw it up.

So what?

Just keep putting in the time and you will begin to become proficient in everything we are talking about here.

Chapter 7: Patterns of Power: Word Strategies

Your Words Contain Power

Everything we are doing to covertly persuade and hypnotically influence someone is about power. The power to influence on an extremely high level is what you are now learning.

Each piece of the pie, each ingredient to the recipe adds up to you being able to pull these technques off masterfully.

As you go through these patterns, you will find some you naturally will love, while others you may not be as fond of. Use "The Grocery Store Approach". When you go to the grocery store, you don't buy everything in the store, you only buy what you need. Do the same thing with these concepts and you'll more out of this than you can ever imagine.

Nominalizatons

Nominalizations are words that take the place of a noun in a sentence, but they are not tangible—they cannot be touched, felt, or heard.

The test for a nominalization is **"Can you put it in a box?"** If a word is a noun and it can't be put in a box, it is a nominalization. Words like *curiosity, hypnosis, learning's, love*, etc. are nominalizations. They are used as nouns, but they are actually process words.

Whenever a nominalization is used, much information is deleted. This is so the meaning is understood by the subject only.

If I say "Johnny has a lot *of "knowledge"* I've deleted what exactly he knows and how he knows it. Nominalizations are very effective in Hypnotic influencing because they allow the speaker to be vague and require the listener to search through their experience for the most fitting meaning.

In the following example, the nominalizations are in bold italics:

"I know that you have a certain *challenge* in your *business* that you would like to bring to a satisfactory *resolution* . . . and I'm not sure exactly what personal *resources* you would find most useful in resolving this *challenge*, but I do know that your *unconscious mind* is better able than you to search through your *experience* for exactly that *resource*. . . ."

In this paragraph nothing specific is mentioned, but if this kind of statement is made to someone with whom you are trying to persuade, he will provide specific personal connotation for the nominalizations used. By using nominalizations, you can provide useful instructions without running the risk of saying something that runs counter to the listener's internal experience.

www.mindforcesecrets.com

Unspecified Verbs

No verb is completely specified, but verbs can be more or less specified. They mentally get them to think of exactly what you want to get across.

If you use relatively unspecified verbs, the listener is again forced to supply the meaning in order to understand the sentence.

> **Words like:**
>
> **Do, Fix, Solve, Move, Change, Feel, Wonder, Think, Sense, Know, Experience, Understand, Remember, Become Aware Of, etc., are relatively unspecified.**

The sentence "I ***think*** this is true" is less specified than "I ***feel*** this is true." In the latter sentence, we are informed as to how the person thinks. If I say, "I want you to ***learn,***" I am using a very unspecified Verb, since I'm not explaining how I want you to learn, or what specifically I want you to learn about what.

Unspecified Nouns

This means that the noun being talked about is not specified.

> "***People*** can succeed."
>
> "***This*** can be easily taught."
>
> "You can notice a ***certain awareness***"

Statements like these give the listener the opportunity to easily apply the sentence to themselves in order to understand it.

Erasure

This category refers to sentences in which a major noun phrase is completely missing.

For example "I know you are ***curious***."

The object of that sentence is missing completely. The listener does not know what he is supposedly curious about. Again, the listener can fill in the blanks with whatever is relevant in his experience.

Creating Strong Cause and Effect Patterns

Everything you are being taught is specifically designed to get you an outcome which you create in your mind. The next section covers some of the most powerful words in order to create a strong "Cause Then Effect".

Example: "When you do that, this happens"

Simple concept, but one that will take you time to embrace, so you can get all of the concepts down.

Linking Words

Using words that imply a cause and effect relationship between something that is occurring and something you want to occur, requests the listener to respond as if one thing did indeed "cause" the other. There are three kinds of linkage, with varying degrees of strength.

- The weakest kind of linkage makes use of conjunctions to connect otherwise unrelated phenomena.

"You are listening to the sound of my voice, **and** you can begin to relax."

"You are breathing in and out **and** *you* are curious about what you might learn."

- The second kind of linking makes use of words that use a connection in time to create powerful strategies to get people to come to your way of thinking based on what they want. Here are some examples:

> **Linking Words:**
>
> As, Before, During, Early, Second, Chief, Former, After, Later, Highest, Another, Was, When, Until, Other, Earliest, Currently, Foremost, First, Along With, Latest, While, Continue, Eventually, In Addition To, More.

*"**As** you sit there smiling, you can begin to see how I can help you."*

"**While** you listen to me speak, you can relax more completely."

Cause & Effect Linking Words:

www.mindforcesecrets.com

> ## Cause & Effect:
> Allows, Forces, Makes, Causes, Requires Creates, Derives, Invokes, Verifies, Justifies, Stimulates, Determines, Bring to Pass, Constitutes

*"Just listening to my offer will **cause** you to want me as your business partner."*

*"Once you **allow** yourself to easily __see the potential of this offering__ you will be able to __make the right decision__".*

Notice that when using each kind of linking word, you will begin with something that is already happening and connect to it something you want to occur. You will be most effective when you begin with the weakest form of linking words and gradually move to a stronger one.

These forms of Linking Words work by implying or stating that what is currently happening will cause something else to occur, and by making a measured transition for the listener between what is happening and some other experience.

The Power of Because

It has been proven that the word "because" elicits a natural response that allows you to get what you are seeking. Most people see the word because as a reason to do something..

Q: Why won't you do the dishes for me?

A: Because

We have all heard variations of that. It is used in business, at home and everywhere else. How many times have you heard someone say?

"Why won't you do it"? – "Because, I just don't want to"!

And most of the time it is accepted. This is the power of because. When combined with a reason that you develop for your suggestion, it becomes a super-powered knockout combination to use for hypnotic influence.

*"When you **see the value** of this truly remarkable product, you will want to **buy it immediately** because it has everything that you have always wanted."*

Now I will add another layer to an already powerful statement (with slight changes)

*"When you **see the value** of this truly remarkable opportunity, you will want to **get involved immediately because** it will allow you to get the things in life you want, and when you do this, it is going to make you **feel real good**"*

Mind Reading

Acting as if you know the internal experience of another person can be an effective tool to build your credibility as long as the mind reading makes use of generalized language patterns.

If the mind reading is too specific, the communicator runs the risk of saying something counter to the listener's experience, and thereby losing rapport.

"You may be wondering what I'll say next."

"You're curious about how I can help you."

Missing Person

An evaluative statement in which the person making the evaluation is missing from the sentence is called a "Missing Person" pattern. Statements using Missing Person can be an effective way of delivering presuppositions, as in the examples, which follow.

"It's good that you can relax so easily."

"It's not important that you sink all the way down in your chair."

Limited Variables

Words such as ***all, every, always, never, nobody,*** etc., are Limited Variables, These words usually limits the variables of a proposition.

"And now you can go ***all*** the way into a trance."

*"**Every** thought that you have can assist you in going deeper into a trance."*

Lack of Choice Words

These are words such as ***should, must, have to, can't, won't***, etc. that indicate lack of choice. These are commands, where you are not giving them an alternative choice.

43

www.mindforcesecrets.com

"Have you noticed that you *can't* open your eyes?"

Chapter 8: The Supremacy of Presuppositions

What Presuppositions Are

Presuppositions are the most powerful of the language patterns to use when you don't want what you have presupposed to be questioned.

Presuppositions are the most powerful word patterns that can be used as they presuppose an outcome. This is how you will control the tempo of a conversation, by determining up front the outcome you want and then putting together the right presuppositions for the situation.

The way to determine what is presupposed and not open to question in a sentence is to negate the sentence and find out what is still true. The simplest kind of presupposition is existence. In the sentence "Bill drove the car" it is presupposed that "Bill" and "car" exist. If you negate the sentence and say "No, Bill didn't drive the car" the fact that Bill and the food exist is still not questioned.

> "A general rule is to give the person lots of choices, and yet have all of the choices presuppose the response you want."

Examples of specific kinds of presuppositions that are particularly useful in hypnotic influencing work follow.

Secondary Clauses of Time

Such clauses begin with words such as

> **Secondary Clauses of Time:**
> Before, After, During, As, Since, Prior, When, While, etc.

"Do you want to sit down *while* you go into trance?"

This directs the listener's attention to the question of sitting down or not, and presupposes that she will go into trance.

" **Before** you sign this contract, would you like something to drink"?

Presupposes that you will sign the contract.

"**After** you get involved with me, you will feel real good about it"

This is where you are bringing the person into the future, presupposing that they will get involved with you and will feel good about it.

"I'd like to discuss something with you *before* you complete this project."

This presupposes that you will complete this project.

Numeric Indicators

> ### Numeric Indicators:
> Another, First, Second, Third, etc. indicate order.

"You may wonder which side of your body will begin to relax *first*."'

This presupposes that both sides of your body will relax; the only question is which will be first.

The Use of "Or"

The word "or" can be used to presuppose that at least one of several alternatives will take place.

*"Would you like to do this now **or** as soon as you are ready?"*

This presupposes that you will do this now or when you are ready. You are ready being a command.

45

*"Would you rather brush your teeth before **or** after you take a bath?"*

This presupposes that you will take a bath and brush your teeth; the only question is in what order.

Awareness Predicates

Awareness Predicates:

Realize, Notice, Think, Speculate, Accomplish, Weigh, Aware, Feel, Perceive, Fulfill, Consider, Know, Wonder, Discover, Grasp, Assume, Understand, Puzzle, Experience, Reconsider, Conceive, Do, Fix, Solve, Move, Change, Think, Sense, Understand, Remember, Become Aware Of

These words can be used to presuppose the rest of the sentence. The only question is if the listener is **aware** of whatever point you are making.

"Do you **realize** that your unconscious mind has already begun to learn...."?

"Did you **know** that you have what it takes to do this successfully?"

"Have you **noticed** the striking effect this program has on your unconscious"?

Adverbs & Adjectives

Such words can be used to presuppose a major clause in a sentence.

Adverbs & Adjectives:

Some, Naturally, Easily, Obviously, Finally, All, Readily, Still, Most, Many, Infinitely, Already, Deeply, Curious, Truly, Begin, Unlimited, Repeatedly, Truly, Accordingly, Usually

www.mindforcesecrets.com

*"Are you <u>curious</u> about how **<u>you can rely on me</u>**"?*

This presupposes that you can rely on me; the only question is it you are curious about it or not.

*"Once you get to know me, you will <u>naturally</u> begin to **<u>feel really good about this</u>?"***

This presupposes that you will get to know me, and that it will naturally feel good to you.

"How *easily* can you begin to **relax around me**?"

This presupposes that you can relax around me; the only question is how easy it will be.

Change of Time Verbs and Adverbs

Change of Time Verbs & Adverbs:
Begin, End, Stop, Start, Continue,
Proceed, Already, Yet, Still, Anymore, etc.

You can *continue* to **enjoy speaking with me**."

This presupposes that you are already enjoying speaking to me.

"Are you *still* interested in getting involved in business with me?"

This presupposes that you were interested in getting involved in business with me in the past.

www.mindforcesecrets.com

Commentary Adjectives & Adverbs

> Commentary Adjectives & Adverbs:
>
> Fortunately, Naturally, Luckily,
> Innocently, Happily, Necessarily, etc.

*"**Fortunately**, there's no need for me to know the details of what you want in order for me to help you get it."*

*"**Naturally**, you will begin to <u>**see the value**</u> of what I am saying to you right now"!*

*"**Luckily**, you have met me today, because <u>**I can help you**</u> with that situation"*

This presupposes everything after the first word.

> **"Stacking many kinds of presuppositions in the same sentence makes them particularly powerful. The more that is presupposed, the more difficult it is for the listener to unravel the sentence and question any one presupposition. "**

Some of the presupposition sentences listed above contain several kinds of presuppositions, and those sentences will be more powerful. The following sentence is an example of the use of many presuppositions stacked together.

*"**Naturally**, as you start to realize the unlimited ways you can **easily** become aware of how using my advice will help you to **truly** accomplish your goals more rapidly and effectively as it relates to your projects, you'll start imagining the success you can **actually** achieve with my help and guidance"*

*"And I don't know how soon you'll <u>**realize the benefits**</u> of this program, because it's not important that you know before you've **comfortably** continued the process of learning these powerful concepts.*

48

Responsive Questioning

Responsive Questioning are yes/ no questions that typically bring out a response rather than a literal answer.

For example, if you approach someone on the street and ask, **"Do you have the time?"** the person generally won't say "yes" or "no."

She will tell you what time it is.

If you ask someone **"Do you know what's on TV tonight?"** it's likely that she will tell you the evening's programming rather than say "yes" or "no.'"

To make Responsive Questions:

1. *You first think of the response you want*. As an example, let's say you want someone to close the door.

2. **The second step is to identify at least one thing that must be true if that person shuts the door.** In other words you are identifying what your outcome presupposes. In this case it presupposes (a) the person is able to shut the door, and (b) the door is now open.

    3. **The third step is to take one of these presuppositions and turn it into a yes/no question.** "Can you shut the door?" "Is the door open?" You now have a question that will typically get you a response without directly asking for it.

Multiplicity of Meaning

This occurs when one sentence, phrase, or word has more than one possible meaning.

> "Multiplicity of Meaning is an important tool that can result in a mild confusion and disorientation which is useful in inducing altered states."

www.mindforcesecrets.com

Anytime you can makes it possible for the listener to internally process a message in more than one way, you require the person to actively participate in creating the meaning of the message, which increase the probability that the meaning will be appropriate for them.

In addition, it is likely that one or more of the meanings wil remain at the unconscious level. The first four patterns described in this document (Nominalizations, Unspecified Verbs, Unspecified Nouns, and Erasure) all function to increase the multiplicity of meaning of the message.

Sounds Alike-Different Meaning

Words that sound alike but have different meanings create another way that causes the person to have to process what you are actually saying either consciously or unconsciously.

> **Such words include:**
>
> - **Right/ Write/ Rite**
> - **I / Eye**
> - **Insecurity / In Security**
> - **Red / Read**
> - **There/ Their / They're**
> - **Weight/ Wait**
> - **Knows/ Nose**
> - **Here/ Hear**
> - **Buy/ By**
> - **Your Mind/ Your Mine**

The following words similarly have two meanings, although they both sound alike and are spelled alike: *left, duck, down, light*. Other examples are: ***push, pull, point, touch, rest, nod, move, talk, hand, and feel.***

Words that have more than one meaning can be marked out and combined with other words to form a separate message. For example:

www.mindforcesecrets.com

"*I* don't know how ***close*** you are to understanding ***now*** the meaning of trance."

The message marked out can be heard as ***"eye close now"***

Extended Sentence

This kind of pattern is created by putting two sentences together that end and begin with the same word.

"*I know that this is something **you will like me**, enjoy it.*" Here the word "like" is the end of the first sentence,

Quotes

This pattern involves making any statement you want to make to another person as if you are reporting in quotes what someone else said at another time and place.

"*As you begin to see the value of this proposition, you will come to the same conclusion that a customer came to the other day, and that was to accept this offer and get started immediately*".

Quotes can be used to deliver any message without taking responsibility for the message. Since you are apparently talking about what someone else said at another time, your listener will often respond to the message, but not consciously identify what he is responding to, or who is responsible for the message.

"*I was speaking with a client of mine the other day and he said that he really hates it when someone says that they will investigate a potentially powerful opportunity and then at the last minute they back off. I couldn't agree with him more. Why don't we spend the next 15 minutes talking about how **this opportunity can benefit you and your family**, shall we?*"

"*My friend Mary told me the other day how she really likes it when a man takes control of the situation and allows her to **get to know this person** in a way that causes her to **get totally excited** about the possibilities of being with this person.*"

www.mindforcesecrets.com

Chapter 9: Telling Hypnotic Stories

Everyone Tells Stories

Telling stories is a potent way in which you can get several things across to someone without directly saying it to them It is one of the true secrets to being able to effecively hypnotize covertly and conversationally.

Telling stories will take time setting up. You must think through the points you are looking to get across and what your end goal is.

Experts in sales and marketing say that "facts tell but stories sell"! When you tell someone a story, they can relate to what you are getting across to them and at the same time, you can be doing many things to influence them through suggestion, presuppositions, subliminal commands etc.

It is suggested that you always have a story that you can tell to someone that is specifically designed and will have the following components

- **Subliminal Commands**
- **Presuppositions**
- **Questions**
- **Suggestive Statements**

The following is an example of how to construct a story. The story can be one that you have actually experienced or it can be a fable or you can tell it from a friend's point of view as well.

This is one of the most powerful methods of speaking to someone and telling them exactly what you want them to hear. The story can be set up several different ways, here are a couple:

The key is to have a story thought out ahead of time, and rehearsed thoroughly. There are so many combinations that I couldn't contain them all here, but use your imagination…

Take your real life experiences and create a subliminal story. Here are some examples of where you can get ideas for your hypnotic stories

- From your own experiences

- From someone elses experiences

- From a movie

- From TV

- From a Book you read

- From a magazine article

- From a news paper

www.mindforcesecrets.com

The possibilities are endless when you create a story line. Use your creativity and imagination.

Basic Story

*"You know it is funny you mention Florida. I took my entire family down their last year and we absolutely had a blast. Did you ever notice that sometimes with a new experience, you really **feel compelled** to get the most out of it that you possibly can? Well, we drove down in our van and it was really fun. I had that feeling like**, This is absolutely the best thing you can do right now.***

*I would encourage you to **experience the benefits of this** as well. You will find that you **grow more interested** in what is going on by the minute. With all the new things to see and take in, it is quite euphoric. Each state has a new look to it and as you **get closer to your goal**, you realize that this entire process has caused you to **get more and more excited** about the final destination.*

*When you **get started with this**, you first feel like it might be the wrong decision, but as you investigate it further, you realize that **this is absolutely the right thing**.*

Do you believe we made it to Orlando in under 24 hours? When you get things done before you expected, you really **get a sense of accomplishment**. It is just a matter of being able to **get involved now** in what is right in front of you."

I could go on and on, but you get the picture. Notice all the subliminal references to what I may be looking to suggest to this person. I have kept it as generic as possible, but you can detail it out depending on how you are trying to influence.

This story is easy to follow and is in a very conversational tone. The next one is designed specifically to alter the state and consciousness of the person by telling a story that is so hard to follow that they have to go into a trance just to try and keep up with the story.

The Twisted Story

The Twisted Story is a method to plant different suggestions into someone's mind by telling a story that is very hard to follow. The reason you do this, is to take the persons mind off in different directions while you are actually implanting your commands right into their subconscious.

Check this story out. It is quite silly, hard to follow, yet when done properly achieves the goal of implanting subliminal messages into the mind of your subject.

"Did I ever tell you about my brother, Chris? It seems he was at this golf outing, and he was at the bar called the 19th hole. And the bartender was telling a story about his buddy who had two brothers. One was really good at dealing with people, but the other had problems until he met this guy named Tom.

Tom was one of these guys that ran in a tight circle of people, he really knew what he was going to *do. And what he wanted to do is drive a cigarette boat. He wanted to **do this now**.*

*Did you ever notice that when you use the power of **"your mine" (mind),** you can really accomplish something? Well, this guy was that type of person. Like me your probably wondering where this is all leading, and all I can tell you is that he finally did get to ride that boat and he did **experience the truly wonderful feeling of this**.*

*(pointing to yourself). Have you ever had an experience like that where you are going so fast that you **get excited** and at the same time the experience is so exhilarating that you know that you must **grab this opportunity that is right in front of you?***

Of course the story can go on and on and it does cause the person to go into trance because of all of the places where things are not completed, yet the story moves into a new direction. How does this fit in? Well of course, you have to plan the story out in advance so that it spells out exactly what you want. You set it up like this.

- What do you want to suggest
- Points to get across
- How confusing do you want to make the story
- Tie the story up so that the ending makes logical sense

www.mindforcesecrets.com

Chapter 11: Combining Suggestive Statements and Presuppostions

A Truly Powerful Combination & Strategy

The following are patterns that were put together by combining a "suggestive statement" (in red) with a pattern that contains presuppositions, embedded commands, and others that have been discussed. It is suggested that you take each of these and work on them for your own area of learning suggestive language.

You will notice that most are from a business angle, but I have also thrown in some from the suggestive forms of relationship building. Please note that all embedded commands will be highlighted and underlined as well as having a pause before each one.

These are the top 68 suggestive predicates to use when looking to influence someone. Keep in mind that you will construct your own patterns out of the suggestive statement/question, presuppositions, subliminal commands and others that we have previously covered.

1. After you **come to.... the conclusion** that what I am talking about is exactly what you are looking for, you will naturally realize that I am the person you are looking for…

2. After you've… **Seen the benefits clearly** of how… **I can help you**, you will better appreciate the work that…. **we can deliver** through our process that will allow you to… **take advantage of our experience** and innovation… Wouldn't that be a truly great advantage that you could benefit from?

3. And the more you allow yourself to find out about how **I can help you**...the more… **you will become interested** in finding out how we can naturally be the vendor of choice for you because we have the right people, processes and technology innovation around the world.

4. And as you…**Allow me to help you** with your initiatives, you'll find yourself being able to… **feel real good** about having me to maximize and bring you more value in, a way that will verify your companies objectives.

5. Are you curious about... How… Good it will feel when you **enjoy spending time with me**

6. Are you aware that... Many top companies choose to work with me because **I can enable your sales team** to be more productive while at the same time bringing more revenue in the door.

7. Are you still interested in... Finding out how… **I can help you** with some of your initiatives?

www.mindforcesecrets.com

8. As you hear these words they... Allow you to reflect on what it is that you really want and when you do that you will be able to ...**see the fun** that we can have together because... **The More You Allow Yourself to Get To Know Me The More You Will Be Glad You Did.**

9. As you...Discover how... **I can help you**..You will ...then...be able to... **experience the value** of having me work directly with your best people.

10. As you consider this...**You realize** that naturally we are the type of firm that... **you will want to engage** on your projects just like some of the top companies that we are currently working with have done.

11. Before you think... about whether.... **you want to engage me** for your project, allow yourself to... **reflect on the value** proposition that I will bring to the table.

12. Can you imagine... Having someone that ...**you can really have fun with** as you **get to know and like me better and better.**

13. Can I ask you to... Take a look at what I can bring to the table for your company because once you see how **I deliver value**, **you will want me to help you** with your projects.

14. Can you visualize.....And... **see the benefits clearly** of how... **I can help you** to deliver exactly what it is you are looking for?

15. Can you...**Set up an appointment with me** to see if... **I can help you** with your needs?

16. Can you remember...The last person you interviewed that you hired that really did a great job and was absolutely fantastic In that job? And as you think about that person and what it was about that person that was so special, I want you to feel free to... **allow yourself to reflect** on how I am the same kind of person and draw the same types of conclusions...I really want you to know how excited I am about how... **I can help you**.

17. Could you...**Become aware** that what I have to propose to you is the right thing to do because... **I am** naturally... **the person** that... **you can rely on**.

18. Do you remember when...You said that you needed a firm that can deliver to you on time and under budget? Well based on what you have told me already, I know **I can easily help you** to maximize your time to market and manage your budgetary considerations.

19. Do you...Ever wonder what it will be like to meet a person that can cause you to... **feel really good** and at the same time be funny, energetic and personable?

20. Do you ever...**Feel good now** about how different your life would be when you can make dramatic changes by meeting the right person.. **Like Me**?

www.mindforcesecrets.com

21. Has it ever occurred to you that... Just listening to what I have to say is the obvious choice for you because… **I can help you with your situation**?

22. Have you noticed that... Just thinking about the business we are discussing will naturally cause you to …**get excited** about how we can make a lot of money together.

23. Have you ever wondered...What it would be like to finally get someone that you can rely on to make sure that everything goes smoothly? Once you understand how …**I can help you**, you will realize that… **I am that person**.

24. Have you...Allowed yourself to… **see the benefits clearly** of working with me?

25. Have you ever...Met someone that you immediately had an attraction to that caused you to… **feel real good** about being with this person?

26. How would you feel if...I suggested that we… **get together now** to go over in more detail how…. **I can help** you with your initiatives/situation?

27. How do you know that..What I am saying is exactly what you are looking for? Well, because… **I have the skills** and information that… **you need** in order to become extremely successful.

28. How do you feel when... Someone easily shows you that they are the kind of person that you would enjoy getting to know better and then allow you to naturally enjoy their company because it makes you… **feel real good**?

29. I don't want you to be...Too surprised to find out that… **I am** just… **the person** you were looking for to handle this situation.

30. I want you to learn... About how… **I can help** with your situation and also.. **allow yourself** to… **see the benefits clearly** of this offering.

31. I know **you are curious**...About how fun it would be to… **get to know me better** because you find yourself starting to… **be intrigued by me** and the more you feel curious about that, the more… **you will want to get to know me better.**

32. I wonder if... **You can help me**….I am looking to speak with the person responsible for (   ).

33. I wonder if….After you… **get to know me better** you will want to… **spend more time with me** because once you… **get to know me better** you will be having so much fun that it will allow you to… **totally relax** in front of me.

34. I wonder could you...Allow me to show you exactly how ….**I can easily help you** with your situation and when I do that it will allow you to… **feel real good** about doing business with me.

35. I would like to suggest that...As you naturally are deciding on the right person for the job that you… **reflect back to our meeting** and allow yourself to… **experience the value** that I will

57

bring to your organization and when you do that you will know that…. **I am the right person for the job** and that will cause you to… **feel real good** about your decision to… **select me** for the position/**hire me now**.

36. I want you to bear in mind…That… **my qualifications** for this position are truly… **what you are looking for** as… **I can help** you in ways that will allow you to really **see the benefits of us working together**.

37. I want you to become aware… Of how… **I can help you** with this because once you become aware of how… **I can help you**, you will know that you have made the right decision.

38. I'd like you to pretend that…**I am the solution to your situation** and that as you reflect on that, you will… **come to the conclusion** that what I am saying is in fact exactly what you are looking for.

39. I'm wondering… Have you ever thought about what it would be like to spend time with someone that will allow you to… **feel real good** about yourself when you are with them, and at the same time allow them to truly get to discover your highest values and interests?

40. I'm curious to know…How your other vendors work with you, and as you reflect on that, you can see how **I can help you** even more with your situation as I am someone that you can naturally and easily come to rely on and… **be convinced** that… **I am the right choice** for this situation.

41. If you could…Design the perfect person to be involved with, would they truly be the type of person that you could… **get to know** and really allow yourself to… **open up** to, or would they be the type of person that would naturally cause you want to… **experience the fun and excitement** that this person could offer you.

42. In my experience… I have naturally found that most people that I deal with are happy with me because they can …**easily rely on me**….When you …**engage me for a project** you will already know how… **I can help you** because I will share with you how you can… **experience the benefits** that other people have come to expect from my services and when you do that it will cause you to **feel real good** about doing business with me.

43. Is it that you are… looking for me to do that, because once you… **experience the value** of how… **I can do that**, you will truly begin to understand how… **I can really help you with that**?

44. Is it possible…That you could… **reconsider your decision** on the proposal, because once you allow yourself to… **focus on how I can help you**, you will then begin to discover exactly the immense value that I can bring to the table… Doesn't that make sense?

45. Is it that you have…Someone else to check with for this decision, because I am sure that once you really understand how… **I can help you**, that you might be surprised to find your self wanting to do business with me because of the things I just said.

46. Is it that there is...Is some other underlying reason for not going ahead or can I suggest that you… **re-evaluate what I said** so that you can allow yourself to… **understand better** the value proposition that I have…..And when you do that, you will… **come to the conclusion** that what I said is exactly what you need.

47. It is useful that... You mention that, because once you realize how… **I can benefit your organization**, you can further understand and… **experience the value** of how **I can help you**.

48. It's impossible...To… **make a decision** without allowing me the chance to show you all I can do for your company because once you see how **I can benefit your organization**, you may be surprised to find yourself wanting to… **hire me now**, so that… **I can help you** and the organization meet their objectives.

49. It's good to know that...Someone naturally as friendly and outgoing as you are, would want to…. **get to know me better**, because once you see how…. **I can make you feel so special**, you will want to… **get to know me even better** and the more you do that the more you will want to …**get to know me even better** and that should cause you to… **feel real good** about getting to know me.

50. It's useful that...You bring that up because once you find out how… **I can truly help you with that**, you will **be thrilled** that you have finally found someone that you can rely on for that.

51. It's good that...You like (Activity) because as you allow yourself to **get to know me better** you will find that…. **I am naturally the most fun person to be with** to do that (activity) and as you… **experience the closeness** that we can share doing that activity, you will be able to… **get to know me even better**.

52. It's not important that... You think I'm not your type, because once you… **get to know me**, you will want to… **spend even more time with me**.

53. It's as if...You have gotten the ultimate opportunity to… **take advantage** of what I am offering. Once you allow yourself to …**see the total value** of what I am offering, you will then be able to see that this is the best deal that you have ever gotten for this.

54. People can loosen up easily...Once they…**get comfortable** and… **relax** with the person they are with. As you …**listen to what I say**, you will… **become more interested** in what I have to say because I will naturally cause you to …**become more comfortable and relaxed** than maybe you have ever been before.

55. Perhaps you are...Wondering how… **I can help you** with your situation. Many people… **work with me** because I help them to identify what is important to them and then show them how they can easily achieve what they want, and the more I show you how… **I can help you** the more you will be naturally interested in being able to… **sign this contract**.

56. Perhaps you can...**Tell me** a little bit more about how… **I can help you**, because once I understand how …**I can help you**, I will be able to help you to… **experience the benefits** of my

www.mindforcesecrets.com

offering and when I do that you will easily… **feel very comfortable** about doing business with me.

57. Perhaps you could…Allow me to show you all of the many wonderful ways that you will enjoy spending time with me .

58. Perhaps you're wondering…Exactly how… **I can help you** with your situation. Once you …**experience the value** of how… **I can easily help you** with your situation you will naturally know that… **I have the the skills** that you are looking for.

59. What do you think would happen if... I could naturally show you exactly what it is you are looking for and at the same time allow you to… **see the value proposition** on what I am offering?

60. What would happen if... I can show you some of the benefits that my clients have received by working with me and at the same time allow you to easily… **see the benefits** of how these things will relate to how… **I can help you**. Once I do this you will naturally… **be convinced** that… **I am the person** to help you with your initiatives.

61. What's it like to...Be able to easily get to know someone that is fascinating and at the same time begin to want to know them even better because they are able to make you… **feel so good** just by speaking with them for just a little bit.

62. When you notice... How easily… **I can help you** ...then...You will naturally want me to help you with your situation.

63. Will you...Tell me exactly what you are looking for in a relationship, because just telling me what you are looking for will allow you to then see that …**I am exactly what you are looking for** and when you do that, you will begin to… **feel real good**.

64. Would you...**Help me** to understand your needs a little better so that **I can easily help you** with the many powerful techniques and strategies that I am going to propose to you today.

65. You **come to... The realization** that… **I can help you**, then you can reflect back on how easily you will… **become successful** with the ideas that I am suggesting for you today.

66. You can become aware that...What I am saying is exactly the answer to your situation and that the more you become aware of what I say the more you will naturally come to the realization that… **I am the answer to your situation.**

67. You know about these things...And the more you know about these things the more you will be able to… **see the value** of how… **I can help you** with these things.

68. You will feel...That…**I am the answer to your situation** because as I explain to you how… **I can help you** benefit from my service will allow you to truly see that I have exactly what you are looking for

www.mindforcesecrets.com

Chapter 11: Suggestive Phrases

Suggestive Phrases to Dominate

Here are the phrases without all of the additional commands, linking words, presuppositions. You can take any of these and start to work with them for your own situation.

You may have noticed when I did these in the sentences; I was all over the board from relationships to business to using this to get a job.

Your possibilities are endless. Just find a couple of these that you find interesting and start to use them in your every day life. They will work fantastic with a little effort.

I don't want you to be...

I want you to learn...

I know you are curious...

I wonder if...

I don't know how soon...

I wonder could you...

I would like to suggest that...

I want you to bear in mind...

I want you to become aware...

I can remember...

I'd like you to pretend that...

I'm wondering...

I'm curious to know...

If you could...

In my experience...

Is it that you are...

Is it possible...

Is it that you have...

Is it that there is...

It is useful that...

It's just like...

61

It's impossible...

It's good to know that...

It's useful that...

It's good that...

It's either (A) or (B); which is it...

It's not important that...

It's as if...

After you come to....

After you've...

And the more you (X)...the more you (Y)

And as you...

Are you curious about...

Are you aware that...

Are you still interested in...

As you hear these words they...

As you... ...then...

As you consider this...

Be aware of what you can sense...

Before you think...

Can you imagine...

Can I ask you to...

Can you visualize...

Can you...

Can you remember...

Could you...

Do you think that...

Do you remember when...

Do you...

Do you ever...

www.mindforcesecrets.com

Don't think of...

Has it ever occurred to you that...

Have you noticed that...

Have you ever wondered...

Have you...

Have you ever...

How would you feel if...

How do you know that...

How do you feel when...

People can loosen up easily...

Perhaps you are...

Perhaps you can...

Perhaps you could...

Perhaps you're wondering...

This can be learned easily...

What do you think would happen if...

What would happen if...

What's it like to...

When you notice... ...then...

Will you...

Would you...

You come to...

You are learning to anticipate...

You can become aware that...

You know about these things...

You will feel...

www.mindforcesecrets.com

Chapter 12: Setting Potent Triggers

Setting Potent Triggers- Stmulus Response Conditioning

Have you ever heard a song from when you were back in High School or College, or maybe it was the song that you and a former girlfriend or boyfriend shared?

When you hear the song, a flood of emotions, memories and recollections come back immediately as if you were back in the day. Everyone experiences these "triggers" to stimulus response, but not many understand how you can set them for your own use in the future.

You are going to learn how to attach a meaning (that you create for someone) and reference to something that can be recalled whenever you want. This trigger is designed to enable you get someone back to a place of heightened emotions that you set previously.

You can build these triggers with the following stimuli:

- Music
- Memories
- Physical Touches
- Gestures
- Certain Trigger Words
- People, Places or Things

Components of an Effective Trigger

When you set these post hypnotic suggestions, you will be able to influence for a long time in the future if done properly.

Identify what qualities, states or behaviors you want to embody and then hypnotically access those states and create potent triggers that are mental, physical or both.

Then practice going into those states as a matter of will. You will want to go out and test your triggers to see how well they worked.

Intensity of The State Accessed

A lot of this is state dependent, which means if you can get someone into a certain state and fire off a trigger, they will respond to that same stimulus and achieve the same state as when you first set the triggering mechanism

- Access state fully and intensely.
- Associate into the state.
- Seeing what you are seeing.
- Hearing what you are hearing.
- Feeling what you are feeling.

www.mindforcesecrets.com

Purity of The State

You want to have one specific set of feelings or emotional state, so you can set the trigger within that person both physically or mentally (words, touches, gestures).

Timing of The Trigger

Start the trigger just before the person reaches the peak of the state or experience.

"Everytime you ( ), You will ( )"- The Suggestion

Pair the trigger with the response as it peaks. Hold it for 5-10 seconds if it is physical.

"This is the eperience you will have"

"You are now experiencing X"

"Review The Experiences of X"

Use a Separator State

- Once the response peaks, distract yourself to a neutral state.
- The neutral state isolates the pairing between the peak experience and the trigger from other random experiences and associations.
- This keeps the association unique.

Use a Unique Trigger

A distinct visual, auditory or kinesthetic trigger will usually work. The best response will occur when you reproduce the trigger exactly as you set it up.

Match the visual, auditory and kinesthetic parts of the trigger exactly.

In order to get proficient at setting the post hypnotic suggestion, you will need to put in the proper fight time to receive the desired results.

www.mindforcesecrets.com

Chapter 13: Hypnotic Induction

The following Hypnotic Induction should be done into a recording device so you can play it back to heare how well you are delivering it.

It is also suggested you read it out loud to yourself, so you can grasp the concepts. This book has built all the pieces of the puzzle to help you deliver your own inductions. This is just an example and can be modified by you to get the specific results you so desire.

Hypnotic Induction Script

As you…. **listen to the sound of my voice** you can…. **go into trance** with eyes open or eyes closed. You may…. **feel more relaxed** by closing your eyes. You may also be sitting in a chair or lying down. When you…. **close your eyes now**, you will begin to…. **feel a sense of relaxation** that will allow all tension and negativity to be released from your body.

As you…. **take in a deep breath**, imagine all tension and negative thoughts to leave your body. As you…. **go deeper into relaxation**, you will notice that sometimes your hands feel warmer and the blood flow in your body causes you to…. **feel real warm and comfortable**. This warmth and comfortable feeling allows you to….. **go even deeper into trance.** As you…… **listen to my voice only**, you will begin to …..**ignore all other sounds** in the room. You may still hear the sounds, but you will naturally and easily ignore them so you can…. **focus on my voice**.

The purpose of the commands you will receive, is to…. **relax your body and mind** so that…. **you will accept the special instructions** that I will speak to you about while…. **you are in trance**. These instructions will be only positive and will cause you no harm. As a matter of fact, these instructions will cause you increase your ability to covertly Persuade and Hypnotically influence someone.

Now what you can do, is just take a few seconds now to… **imagine** the kind of place where you could be at this time that would totally cause you to **go deeper into this state of relaxation and trance**. This place is your place. You choose where you are. It can be at the beach, in the forest, or even space. Because you are using your wonderful imagination, you create the place. The place can be a special workshop of the mind, that you have designed. A place where only you can go.

As you see that place, hold it in your mind, but do not go there yet. I want you to imagine a large chalk board in front of you, one like you used to have when you were in school. I want you to take a piece of chalk from the board…. **Focus on the chalk board.**

www.mindforcesecrets.com

I would like you to draw a box on the board, with your brilliant imagination. In that box, I want you to draw a large letter "A". The "A" should fill up the entire box from top to bottom and side to side. Next I want you to draw a letter "B" and do the same thing, making sure that it totally fills the box on the sides and from the top to the bottom. You will do as much of the alphabet as you can slowly and with great concentration, as I count down to the number 10. It is not important that you finish the entire alphabet, but that you….. **focus on what you are doing**. You will focus on writing on the chalk board and even though you will…. **hear my voice**, I want you to…… **concentrate on what you are doing**.

10….You are going ten times deeper than the moment before.

9…. You are relaxed and confident with your persuasion skills

8…..As you go down deeper into trance you realize that your hypnotic power grows stronger every day.

7….Listen to my voice…When it comes to persuading others you are bold and confident at all times.

6…..Relax down deeper because the more you relax, the more you will be able to experience the benefits of this trance.

5… You are 25 times deeper than you were before and this allows you to feel even better about your ability to influence, because you are strengthening your mind on a daily basis.

4… Your voice is naturally becoming a powerful tool that you can use to get people to come to your way of thinking. You know just the right tone to use at just the right time.

3….The strength of your gaze alone, causes people to want to get to know you even better.

2….As you relax down deeper, you begin to feel the confidence that you have always dreamed of.. People are attracted to you because of the magnificent presence that you have.

1… You are now 100 times deeper than before and you are a total controller of every situation in your life.

As you **go into trance even deeper**, I want you now **go that special place** that you created in your imagination. This place can be a place of solace, relaxation and place for you to re charge yourself. Think of it as a mind vacation, a place that you can visit anytime you want…. **You are a controller**, so use this place as a place where you can plan out projects or a place where solutions to situations can be performed.

As you reflect on how…. **you are confident** now, maybe more so than you have ever been before, you can easily…. **see the value of conditioning the mind**. Your mind is your most potent weapon. Now that ….**you are a controller** of all of the circumstances in life…. **you can harness the full power of your mind**. Your powers of persuasion and influence grow stronger each day, because you take the time to increase your knowledge and practice daily. This alone will cause you to…. **feel real good about this**.

www.mindforcesecrets.com

Now, you are going to come out of trance when I count from 1 to 10. When I get to the number ten, I want you to open your eyes and feel refreshed and energized as if you just had the best, most restful sleep of your life. As I count, I want you to…. **feel the energy** in your body starting to increase. I want you to…. **feel the confidence** that comes with this training. I want you to feel the power of being a controller.

1…2…3…4…5…6…7…8…9…10… Open your eyes. You are totally refreshed and energized, bold and confident to take on all of your day's challenges.

www.mindforcesecrets.com

Chapter 14: Manipulation Quick Reference Guide

We've gone through all the info we need to for this course all the info that is pertinent as far as what you need to do in order to get people to the right stages and states and be able to persuade and influence them powerfully. What I want to do now is to do a short review this will be a quick reference guide that you can use in order for you to grasp what you need to do.

I was always the type of person when I went to a training class or a seminar or even listen to a set of audio programs like this, I always thought, I would like to have the information summed up because although the information is good, it is a lot to handle. I am also the type of person that likes to know something right off the bat. I like to get on the ground and start running as soon as possible. That is what I am going to do with the quick reference guide.

This will be a section that you can go back to anytime you need to get a quick reference on what we went over. Of course for any details go back to the coarse, to the notes, go back to the recordings and really dig deep into what's there. But I have laid it out in a way that you should be able to go to the program and you have the backup notes which will correspond to the audio program so that you can really practice as soon as you've gone through the program one time.

Once you go through the program one time, you can go back to the reference material, and go back to the manual and start to actually put this into play. That is the key that we will be talking about is how you put this into play.

Many times I would go to trainings and learn a lot of these things but the instructors never told you the real world applications. They never told you how to get this to work, how to get this into play how to train with these technologies.

This is the key to your success....

It doesn't really do you good if someone gives you a bunch of techniques and says here's a bunch of techniques, go out and use them. You have to know how to use them, when to use them. You have to know technologies on training, just like I mentioned before that just because you know something, doesn't mean that you're skilled at it.

Just because you know how to lift weights, doesn't mean you're in perfect body building fitness. Just because you know how to do martial arts, in terms of some of the punches and kicks, doesn't mean you can pull them off in a serious situation.

What this is intended for as far as the reference guide is to go over many of the concepts we covered so that you can really have in your mind what you need to do when you are looking to persuade, or looking to put someone into a trance like effect, strengthen concentration, exactly what you need to do to go to point A to point B.

Trust + Needs (Reasons) = Action

We talked about getting that trust, moving from the trust to where their needs are, there reasons. Of course having your presentation done and the ultimate is the action that is where we get the results for the hard work we put in. What you need to do is you need to go through the book especially and take a look at things in chronological order. I've put things as much as I could in a chronological order.

www.mindforcesecrets.com

Energy, Intent & Attitude

The first thing you are going to do is the energy and the intent and the attitude. Although this is not a technical piece of information, it really is technical because like I've said many times throughout this program it's your attitude, your belief in your own abilities, it's the intent that you have when you go out to do these skills.

This is what's going to make a difference. I'd rather have a person who believes in themselves and has the intent to go out and do these properly than someone else that has technical skill. I know many guys that have great technical skills, but never used the technical skills.

They can tell you up and down all about the skill but they really cannot go out and do it. Bringing out how you are going to get to do it, you need to go out and do it. If you are going to get good at these skills, you are going to have to get out and practice.

Get Good At Conducting Formal Inductions

We talked a little about doing formal inductions, I would recommend you do that,. If you have a willing accomplice, someone who is willing to sit down with you and go through some trance inductions, you can do it with all the material you have in this course. All you have to do is go through all the different patterns we put together, go through the trance induction that I put together for you that you listened to, build your own trance inductions.

They key to putting together a trance induction is allowing the person to go into trance naturally. Not only in words, but by the pace of the words, by the tone of your voice and also how you put those phrases together.

What is going to be the end result, what is the induction going to do? Is it going to just put the person into a trance? Are you going to tell them a story and put them into a trance? How are you going to conduct the induction, this will take some homework on your part.

You will have to sit there and put together the induction. As you sit there with your eyes closed, relax your body and just go right through the script that I had, you can change it and modify it to what you want to do.

That's a good way to get the tonality down, a good way to get these skills down. When you are doing it this way, that's not conversational at all, but that is where you will start to build up the belief, and your intent. The better you get at it, the better you're going to get at it.

I have had a lot of people who contact me and say, I've tried putting someone into an induction and it didn't work, I said, hey.. it happens to everyone. Not everyone you attempt to do an induction for will work the first time; you might have to do it several times.

I have a friend of mine that is very difficult to get under hypnosis. So you have to really use the techniques I've talked about. You've got to know their personalities, if their not willing to give up that control so you can hypnotize them, they will be very hard subject to hypnotize...

That's why you have to find somebody or some bodies that you can play with and if they want to learn hypnotism, you teach them at the same time. They hypnotize you and you hypnotize them, and you see how deeply you get into the trance. That's probably the best way to do it.

If you don't have a partner like that than you will have to rely on video recording or audio recordings, the easiest way is to use a software like "audacity", recording yourself, and listening how you sound. You do need to get some feedback at sometime, and that's when I recommend you go out

70

www.mindforcesecrets.com

and meet people and you start to use the conversational hypnosis structures in the process of going out and doing your daily things.

I'm not saying you should do it in a way you are going to mess someone over in a shopping mall.

How To Tell If Someone Is In Trance

The ways you can tell someone has gone into their trance. How can you tell if someone is in a trance?

You can tell by their eyes... If their eyes start fluttering a little bit or they kind of get that stare, then you know that they are somewhat going into a trance like state. They have strength of concentration, you can look at them and see that they are concentrating.

You can also tell by the direction they are looking. A lot of times when you ask someone a question they will go back in their head to try and get the answer. Did you ever ask somebody a question, and they knew they knew the answer, but had to retrieve it from the file. So what they will do is look up and think… where was that?

They couldn't remember which, but they go to the file and pull out the information. You could notice some processing while they are thinking about it. When they are thinking about it and processing it, they are in an alternate state.

SO keep those things in mind as we are lining ourselves up to do these patterns and phrases on people.

The Power of The Voice

The power of your voice, working on your voice tone, getting it down as deep as you can. *(Lowering voice)*. This is obviously not my normal voice, but for some people it can be quite entrancing, listen to the sound of my voice and as you listen, it will cause you to go deeper into trance. You're going to have to work with your own voice.

Your speaking voice, when you're speaking to a woman you use the softer tones because they like that and as you use the language we talk about its entrancing. Part of the reason why you would actually get someone to go into a hypnotic type of state is because of the quality of the voice. The voice has a hypnotic quality to it. It draws the subject in...

You speak a little slower and they hold onto every word you say. When you say words that grab an emotional point on them, for instance, you are going to cause them to feel real good. A lot of people do not hear that statement, so when you tell people you are going to cause them to feel good, it brings over the feeling of that....

Anytime you can make someone feel real good, they are starting to be persuaded by you.

By the same token, when you talk to someone about how **you can rely on me**, **you're going to like me**, when they hear that in a soft tone of voice, it's kind of like floating down the river, so relaxing that people just melt like butter listening to your voice.

Work on the voice tone, it's a very important part of this process, you will look a little strange doing it but you want to be able to have the different voice tones so you can monitor it. You will really know what will work best for you. I know some guys that use the more relaxed voice tones and get great results with it. It depends on the personality of the person you are dealing with as well.

71

The Power of The Eyes

Powers of the eyes - always look people in the eyes when talking to them. As you're setting up the trance, you definitely want to be looking in their eyes because your eyes are putting forth a lot of energy so make sure you are putting that energy across.

Always send the energy out to someone. This is part of the belief and attitude, but you always want to be pushing that nice calm energy towards them. You are using this as visualization, but in reality it absolutely goes out to them whether you can see the energy or not, it doesn't really matter, but that energy is going there. Hopefully it is a positive energy.

We are taking somebody down a road and that's what we are really doing with all these concepts. It's like you have entered them into the building with intent and energy and guiding them down this corridor, and as we go down this corridor, we are taking them deeper into this corridor and as we go down, obviously we are sending them good energy and intent. We are using everything that we can in terms of pulling them in. We're using the voice tones to relax them and put them into a certain state. We are now going to be moving into the bonding and rapport...

The Bonding & Rapport Process

This whole process of bonding and rapport and the energy and intent, and the voice, its all being designed and built to get trust. The more somebody trusts you, the more they will give themselves over to you both consciously and unconsciously... It is a wonderful process.

You can't control somebody; they have to give you the control. That's why we are the controllers because we are controlling ourselves, but they are giving us the control... So as we move down this persuasion and hypnotic influence corridor, we are building up the bonding and rapport to do that. We are using all the skills of bonding and rapport to do that.

We are using all the techniques that we have learned, were getting them to know us, to like us and to ultimately to trust us. We know that likes attract, so we are going as close to them as we can. We want to almost be like their twin, we want to know the different personality types, the sharks, the whales, the urchins and the dolphins and understanding how each of those personality types fit into the individuals we are looking at.

The other thing is **matching, mirroring, pacing** them. There is also a thing called verbal pacing and what that does is it will allow you to get to the point where you're actually pacing their reality, but bringing them into yours.

How you're going to do that is pace the reality of the situation you're in. That's why you hear a lot of hypnotists will use a pacing technique. This is where they will reference what is a current reality. You're sitting in a chair, and as you sit in that chair you can feel the fabric of the chair on your hands. And as you listen, you can hear the sirens in the background, they must be going to a fire. And as you reflect on the smell of coffee in the office... That's called pacing the reality. When you do that, it makes the person go into a quasi trance because they are thinking of all of the things consciously that they were already unconsciously aware of.

For instance, when you sit down into a chair, you don't make a reference on those things, the fabric, my feet are touching the floor, oh I hear a siren and then the smell of coffee, you're not doing that. When somebody says that to you, it automatically causes you to reference that information. When you reference that information, you are starting to go into a trance.

72

www.mindforcesecrets.com

Remember, anytime the state is changed, anytime there is strength of concentration, you go into a trance or trance like state.

Secrets of Pacing & Leading

Once you're pacing their reality, you're then going to pace the reality and your then going to pace what you want to get across... This point is your objective, your command. Something like, as you continue to sit there in the chair. You're going to allow yourself to feel so good when you act on my advice. So you are letting them know that just by sitting in the chair they:

1. Feel so good

2. Will act on your advice

So what I did was I paced a couple of times as you continue to sit in the chair and begin to relax even more, that's pacing the reality of the situation. You're going to act on my advice. So I've done 2 paces and then do what I call a lead.

A lead is actually sending an affirmation or a directive at that person. You wouldn't want to do the directive as soon as you get into the situation. You want to pace it first, 3 or 4 or 5 paces and then you want to slip in a lead.

You do a couple 2-3 paces, and then add in 2 leads and then you're going to even it up so there is an equal amount of paces as there are leads and then what you're going to do is your going to lead the entire time., you are actually going to start bombarding them in their consciousness with what you want them to know.

Pace: As you sit there listening to the sound of my voice

Pace: You can smell the coffee, hear the sirens and feel the fabric of the chair

Lead: As you do that you will start to feel real good and act on my advice

Lead: When you act on my advice, you will feel real good

Lead: When you feel real good, you can start to experience many wonderful things

So you have relaxed them down, set the frame for them and then you're going to hit them with the directives that are called pacing and leading. It is an important concept to understand. It is something you can keep in your head as your putting this information together, it works specifically in the bonding and rapport area. As your getting the bonding down, you're not only pacing them physically, your also going to bond by doing all the matching and everything that goes along with that.

So that's the key you need to look for in the bonding and rapport and building that relationship with them so they feel like you're their best friend from 20 yrs ago. That's the key to building up the bonding and rapport, just making yourself up so much like that person, that they enjoy begin around you.

Needs & Intents = Powerful Motivation

So you've gotten the trust to a certain level, now you need to find out what their needs are, what their intent is. This is a very important part because you now have to find out what motivates them, what is their motive, what is going to be their motive for you to get your point across. It is an excellent strategy to do this; you can look at it from any perspective. We as human beings are looking at every

73

www.mindforcesecrets.com

situation for our benefit. They say when someone hands you a picture of a group with everyone in it and you, you always look for yourself first.

Because we are focused on ourselves, we really have our own agenda for what we want to accomplish. So even though I am trying to persuade somebody, I really need to have an idea of how this will benefit them because if it is just going to benefit me, it will be a lot harder to actually get them to do what I want them to do.

You can get them to perceive that it will benefit them, but in my opinion it is misleading and unethical. All you need to do is to find out what their motivation is, and plug in the motivation. Plug in all the information they need in the way you can help them with the particular situation.

So if they are motivated to buy your product because it's going to help them, whatever way that is, they basically give you the information you need and spit it back at them. If they tell you they are looking for something that will increase their health, and that's the kind of product you have, you go back and say, hey I am glad you said that because that is one of the strong features of our product, is that it really benefits the health and I think that you will see based on what you just said that this is the product for you.

Or if it's a person in a relationship situation, I've always looked for someone who is caring and trustworthy, you take that and spin it right back at them. I am glad you said that because as you sit here and talk to me, you'll discover that I am very caring and trustworthy. Again you are using a quotes pattern to use this information to throw back at them. So you have your reasons and your needs. We've gotten the trust, the reason, they are beginning to put their arms around us and are kind of becoming their buddy.

Creating Powerful Embedded Commands

We are going to move into the presentation facet. The presentation facet will have a lot of different things. The best way to go into the presentation is that you now have their reasons and motivations, you need to determine what yours are...

What are your embedded commands going to say, what is it ultimately want to get out of this person?

The way you look at an embedded command, you take away all the sentences, all of the information that we've talked about up to know, take away all the rapport and bonding you have to build and think as if you can merely go up to someone and request something –

"Give me $100 dollars"

"Here is my product, buy it now and write me a check".

If it was that simple to make the sale, then that would be what you would say, you wouldn't have any of the idle chit-chat.

You would go to everyone on your block, or you would go to every office complex and you would sell the product, or go up to everyone of the opposite sex and you would contact them, "hey, I would like to go out with you, give me your phone number, let's go out tomorrow night, we'll go to dinner - you'll pay for it, so on…"

The reality is that we know that it does not work that way. But when you're looking at it in an embedded command, you're looking in a subliminal directive that is in essence exactly what you're doing with those directives.

74

The Directive is Exactly What You Want to Happen

It is as if your saying to them those directives, so when your building up your entire sentence structure, the embedded command is what your shooting across. What is the delivery mechanism for the embedded command?

The delivery mechanism for the embedded command is a lot of the other word phrases that you have learned up until now. They are used with very specific purpose and that's why we use them.

It is a lot of the other ways we are going to delivery those embedded commands, through presuppositions and other methods. Remember those are phrases that are going to presuppose that what we are going to say are, correct and what they need to do that moment in time. We're putting this all together for their benefit. We're also using the suggestive phrases.

We are also going to work on, as we are putting our presentation together, comeback lines, in case someone gives us a smart response or remark or some type of look...

You have to have a comeback line. So you want to have 5 comeback lines that you can say to somebody if they reject your idea. That's how you're going to work on it.

Of course we have gone through all those phrases, so you can go back and go through those sections, but this is how we are aligning them. This manual has a lot of this information, so you can go back and start to put together your game plan of how you're going to persuade.

Putting in The Proper Flight Time

When you first go out, let's say you want to do this in public and you go to the library and you're going to start pulling off patterns with somebody. The first way you're going to start doing it is your going to go up to them and meeting them, and then what you're going to do is start saying a few little things.

You're going to try some directives, some very simple things. Then you are going to test it, you're always testing. Now maybe that's the first day, maybe the second day you go out and try some more. I wouldn't recommend that you take all of this information that you've gotten here in the course and try and memorize it, and go out there and try and deliver it.

I tried it in the beginning and it is very difficult and you sound foolish. Unless you really put in the flight time which if you do put in the flight time, then go and give it a shot. You want to bite size this process, do little bits and pieces, you want to get comfortable with it, and you want to stay away from as much negativity as you can.

In the beginning you may get some people that look at you with these eyes that say what are you talking about? So if you do it the right way, they will never even know you are using these skills on them, they will say talk more, they like what you're talking about, especially if you're weaving in stories, you're weaving in the quotes pattern.

Remember to Use the Quotes Pattern

The quotes pattern can be used for any number of reasons as I mentioned a little while ago. Using the quotes pattern, allows you to have trustworthiness with the people you are influencing So if you find out somebody's reason, you use that and sling it back at them in a context that will bring light into what you are doing.

www.mindforcesecrets.com

Again you want to use this as ethically as you can. I would never use these skills to try and harm somebody, and in my opinion if you do, you will get what's coming to do.

There are people who abuse everything that's out there from guns to using their fists, and this is very strong, very powerful techniques and combination that you can be messing with somebody's mind.

So you don't want to do it in a way that you're going to harm them. You don't want to do it in a way that you're slipping in these embedded commands that are just not right. I've heard of people that have done that personally, I have never been associated with people who have done that, and hopefully I never will. The main thing is to keep these things as ethical and as pure as you can.

Focus on The Process

One of the key things when you're doing the word patterns or word phrases, sentence phrases, is really understanding that it's not so much the content of what you're saying, it's the process your putting them through. And the process is the entire thing that we are talking about. So if you're looking at things in terms of a process, not just the content you're putting out there, you're going to get much better results because the process is your weaving the entire process through the conversation that you're using.

You might be using a few presuppositions, you've got embedded commands, you might have a story you slip in that you use all the time that says something. Let me give you a few that I think work right off the bat that you can start working with.

"What if" is a powerful statement, it creates a very good imaginative state. it gets their imagination going. *What if you can find the exact person that could help your company go to the top. That really creates an imaginative process, especially for a company that is looking for someone to take them to the top in their industry.* The same for a relationship. *What if you could find the person that you've always dreamed of,* it brings up all kinds of imagination of what that person could be, so it's a very good trance type phrase. Of course you got to have stuff behind it to be able to peel into it.

"The More" *The more you find out about me, the more you will like me*. That is a very powerful one; you can work in as well. *What if you can find somebody that you are really attracted to, not only because of the way they look, but because the way they treated you, and they made you feel so good, and you found out that the more you dealt with this person, the more you knew, the more you really found that they were the exact type of person you were looking for.*

So basically what I did was combine both of those into a sentence phrase that you can actually use. A lot of people say when you are doing these sentence phrases; it's not really a 2 way conversation. That's the trick of getting this down naturally.

Everything takes time and being bold and confident with what you are doing.

Learn How to Evaluate Your Skills (Self Evaluation)

At first you will be very robotic, you will go out there and you're going to be thinking, again you're rehearsing your lines, you're an actor, and so your thinking of the lines, after you get it down good enough, the lines will come naturally. You've done them so many times that when somebody says something, you respond, you have a comeback.

www.mindforcesecrets.com

You're going to realize that once you start this technology and you get somebody to a trance stage and you'll say something that will pull them totally out. You'll say what did I do wrong?

You will look back at it and recognize what you did wrong, I didn't stay on this one point, you kind of diverted and pulled them out of the entire state. I can't really teach you those things; you have to learn them as you go through the process. Every situation will be different. I know when I talk to people; I make notes in my head of what I did right and what I did wrong.

Sometimes you go through and it just flows right through, it just rolls right off your tongue and you get the results you are looking for. It's a matter of action; it's a matter of going out there and putting this into action. Let me talk about a few things that I did not get a chance to cover in the actual course.

You Have to Be Covert When Talking to Those You Know

When you start to talk like this, people will start to look at you differently because they realize that you are talking differently than you did before. But this is something you can turn on and off. Obviously if you're hanging out with your buddies, you're not going to be talking in a trance language with them or they will think you are a little weird...

When I first starting doing this, and started talking to my wife and trying to pull patterns on her, she wasn't buying it at all, so I had to be a lot more covert when I was doing things because she knew it. She knew how I talked and all of a sudden I slowed down my tone of voice and I have a different voice, she said, hey why are you doing this, you sound crazy.

But for someone who doesn't know me that well, I can put on that type of voice and it totally entrances them, they totally dig it. So when you're first getting started, you have to keep all these factors in mind so you can really embrace it.

I also talked about increasing your vocabulary, increasing your words. Part of the reason you are putting people into a trance like state just by using certain words, or word phrases is that they may have never heard anyone speak like that before, and it's like your speaking in a romance type language, in a sense that it is a very visual type of language, its language that really elicits a response from them not only physically but also elicits a response from them going into the brain and process the information you are giving them.

Whether you are talking to a male or female doesn't really matter, but I will say that females will pick up on the information and the energy that you are sending a lot better because they are in more trance by that type of language, the kinder, nicer type of language patterning. There are certain words that you can use, that I call power words. Now these aren't words that are necessarily trancing words, but are words that you can use that are powerful when writing and speaking.

You can use these words and you will see these words in the book. They are words like adapt, analyze, and collaborate on. A lot of these words are used in a business context, but you can use them in the relationships too. Cultivate, how would you like to cultivate a relationship with somebody. When you say cultivate, it is something they don't hear every day so they have to process it.

- Harness
- Enhance
- Familiarize
- Foster
- Navigate

77

www.mindforcesecrets.com

- Initiate
- Interpret
- Leverage
- Nurture
- Persuade
- Quadruple
- Streamline
- Synthesize
- Target
- Traction
- Triple
- Velocity
- Smoothness

Any descriptive words that you can find, that why when I say when you are looking up words to find the most descriptive words that you can. Anytime you get a descriptive word and use it, it is a listening and response based on their reference. So if you say if we did this with smoothness, they are interpreting this smoothness as what they know as smoothness. You don't have to explain that, you are being vague, but using a word that is outstanding.

Take these words, and start to intermingle them in your tool box of what you are doing. Also the course has jammed packed more information than you can use right now. There is really too much information in the course. I tried to cut it down as much as possible, but I knew I had to give you as much as you needed and I don't think it's an over kill, maybe it's an over skill. You will have enough information so that you can go back to it.

I really want to reference and really emphasize the fact that you want o go into the section where you have the suggestive phrases and sentences and you want to take those beginning part of those sentences, the "if you could", the "as you" and all of those types of phrases and start finding out your top 10 or top 20. There are just under 70 of those phrases. So you want to take the top 10, the ones you like, the ones that you can pull out of your pocket, no problem any time of day. Those are the ones you will start with and you will start putting together patters.

Hypnotic Influence Works, When You Work It

You will take your embedded commands and you start putting those in, then the presuppositions, just a couple of those words and put those in like naturally, luckily, easily and put those in. this is how you are getting started using the technology. You are taking it one bite at a time. You're not trying to take the course as a totality and saying, ok I have to understand everything because you don't need to understand everything, you just need to understand the things you need right now, and that is getting started.

A lot of people look at this information and say hey, I'm not going to go out there and try to persuade or hypnotically influence somebody until I got these techniques down. My point is if you never go out and try, you will never make it. First, you don't try you only do. Your attitude has to be

78

that you are not trying to do this, you are doing this. When you go out, you are the controller and you are going to influence somebody. You have to get in your head that you are in control of the situation. You have to go out there and keep practicing.

Like the guy that came up to me and said I tried to do an induction and it didn't work. I told him you did one somebody or 100 somebody's? He said 1 somebody a friend of mine; I said well, so what? There are going to be some that are going to actually grasp onto what you are doing, others won't.

I had one guy that came to me and said I cannot be hypnotized. I said have a seat, were just going to talk, forget all this hypnotizing stuff, it's kind of crazy don't you think, he said yeh, absolutely. I just started talking to him, telling him a story and started embedding some commands and things like that.

A couple of day later he said to me, what were we talking about the other day, I feel different, it was just so strange the way you were talking to me. I said well I said it's because I hypnotized you, he said get out of here, and I said absolutely, it was conversational hypnosis because you already told me that you could not be hypnotized. So I had to not even mention it, so if you mention it to some people, they will resist it.

Conversational Hypnosis Is Power

That's why conversational hypnosis is so powerful. Your kind of going through the back door, talking to them naturally and doing all the trance stuff and they think you are doing what you normally do but you got your embedded commands in there and your little phrases, and words and comebacks and everything is really neat and by the end of the situation you got them to do exactly what you wanted them to do.

At the end, they are shaking their hand and their happy as can be, they don't even know what is going on. But you've done it in a win-win situation, their fired up, and excited that they came to some decision or you did something exactly the way you wanted to do it.

That's what conversational hypnosis is, you're not going to get them to bark like a dog or cluck like a chicken. There just going to do what you ask them to do because you are embedding the commands, and when you embed the commands strong enough it will work. Take this information and really utilize it, work with it every day, take a few minutes out of you day. Look at the scripts, look over the different patterns, figure out your favorite embedded commands and start working with them.

As you start working with these, you are going to notice down the road that you're going to get more powerful with your words, and your patterns and will find out that you are the controller of your life and that as you become a stronger controller, you begin to allow others to give control over to you. So that you can help them, so that you can help them see the benefits of how you can help them. And when you do that, you are going to get the most and maximum out of life that you've gotten.

If there are any questions on this course, if there is any information on this course you would like to discuss just give me a call or email me, I would be more than happy to answer any questions you may have. Good luck and keep persuading.

www.mindforcesecrets.com

Chapter 15: Glossary of Concepts

Presuppositions - A statement or question that presupposes something or things have to be true in order for the statement to make sense. Stack presuppositions together but only use when you have already created a trance state otherwise they will have little to no effect.

Mirroring - Matching Externally the subjects vocal qualities, breathing, posture, physical gestures,. Matching internally their values, beliefs, attitudes, etc. by eliciting those and stating agreement with those aspects. Matching a person's breathing and speaking at the same rate creates an incredible sense of Rapport and gives you the ability to lead them in the direction of your outcome.

Quotes - Stating what another person said to you as a way to create that state in your subject. "The other day one of my customers said this is the very best product in the world". By using the quote, you can use a third party to endorse what you are saying. Also can be used to say something directly to someone without them realizing your speaking to them.

Values Hierarchy - Eliciting their values in a business,relationship, ranking them in order, stating them in order back to them thereby creating, an intense euphoric state and linking that state to yourself with physical gestures and linking commands. This allows everyone you come in contact to pick up the good feelings from you.

Tonality - Making your tonality match the state you are working to elicit. And also dropping your voice (commanding) to mark out certain words and/or phrases to bypass the conscious mind and deliver messages (embedded commands) to the subconscious mind of the subject or client.

Embedded Commands - Commands hidden inside of sentences and marked out by a change in voice tone or physical movement and meant to deliver those commands to the subconscious mind without the awareness of the conscious mind.

Personal Trance Words – A subjects own personal highly emotional trance state triggering words. Elicited by asking questions that elicit a deep trance state to answer and then fed back using specific language to influence them even more.

Reinforcer - "you know how the other day we were talking about how you can feel an incredible ..."

Binder Commands - To me, Do it, Now, With me, Experience that, Taking place now, etc.

Triple Verification - Quote an Article or Show, then a friend, then give your opinion.

Distortion of Time - "Imagine a time in your future", "Looking back on it, or this"

www.mindforcesecrets.com

Installing Your Voice In Their Head - "You say this persons words, as if their words are your internal voice ..." or "that special place in your mind, where you know what's true, you hear that voice that's true (your voice of course)"

Amplifier - "and you're probably not aware how when you make those pictures bigger and brighter, how the feelings get much more intense ..."

Perspective - "you just start to look through a different set of eyes" or "you see things in a whole new way ..."

Negation - "you really shouldn't, it's not necessary, don't find yourself, don't think about, etc.

Adjectives - Incredible value, Overwhelming attraction, Uncontrollable desire, Powerful, Unbelievable, Intense, Undeniable, etc.

"NOW" - Orients them in the now to do it now, not later.

"STOP" - Makes the subject stop their internal process or interrupts it, so you can put things in.

Post Hypnotic Suggestions - To make the subject think about you when you are not around and re-experience states you have already elicited. Link those states, representations to common things that happen to them but not things that happen all the time.

Focus Blending - Listen carefully, hang on every word, the rest of the environment disappears, fades away, really pay close attention, a certain aspect of his face starts to rivet your attention, listen to the sound of his voice, find that you can picture it clearly, etc.

Reality Stacking - Telling a story inside of a story inside of another story so her conscious mind can it keep up with what is what part of what story so it gives up.

Embedded Questions - Bypasses resistance, also creates,, response potential. "I'm wondering whether you realize what a incredibly amount of value you will derive from having me head up your projects"

Push & Pull - When you get them going in one direction, something pulling them as well as pushing them in your direction.

Chapter 16: Other Resources

When I wrote this book originally back in 2001, I wrote is as notes for myself. Over the years, the Manipulation course has sold the world over and is one of the most popular Hypnosis Study courses on the planet. This all started with me making notes for myself to help myself get better.

This updated edition has about 3 times the amount of content as did the original manuscript. I am proud of the information and know you will get a great deal of knowledge by applying the principles in this book.

Here is a look at some of the other books and or courses I have written with the websites, so you can get more information.

www.mindforcesecrets.com

- Closed Door Hypnosis Files

- Manipulation

- Internal Power Centers

- Magneto

- Mind Portal

- Goal Setting Fomula

www.chipower.com

-Chi Power Plus

- Mind Portal

- Internal Power Centers

- Advanced Chi DVD

- Chi Power Inner Circle Membership

www.mindforcesecrets.com

www.mindforcesecrets.com